So Far Away

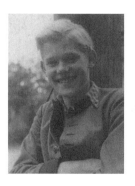
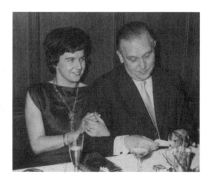

So Far Away

A Daughter's Memoir of Life,
Loss, and Love

CHRISTINE W. HARTMANN

Vanderbilt University Press
Nashville

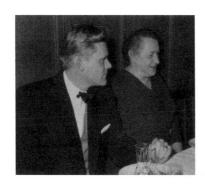
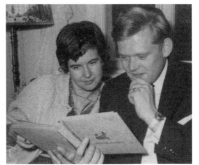

© 2011 by Vanderbilt University Press
Nashville, Tennessee 37235
All rights reserved
First printing 2011

This book is printed on acid-free paper.

Library of Congress Cataloging-in-Publication Data

Hartmann, Christine W.
So far away : a daughter's memoir of life, loss,
and love / Christine W. Hartmann.
p. cm.
ISBN 978-0-8265-1795-1 (cloth edition : alk. paper)\
ISBN 978-0-8265-1796-8 (pbk. edition : alk. paper)
1. Hartmann, Christine W. 2. Hartmann, Christine
W.—Family. 3. Adult children of aging parents—
United States—Biography. 4. Mothers and
daughters—United States—Biography. 5. Fathers
and daughters—United States—Biography. 6. Aging
parents—Care—United States. 7. Terminal care—
United States. I. Title.
HQ1063.6.H374 2011
306.874092—dc22
[B]
2011003062

To
Antje
and
Ron

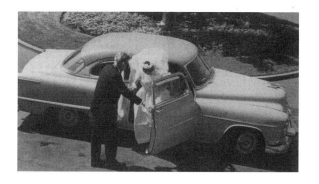

Irmgard:

"I have always been scared of death. But now that I've decided I'm not going to leave that final event to chance, I feel much better. I can be in control of it, and this gives me a kind of inner peace nothing else can."

"Wait. Please listen to me. I don't want you to do it!"

"Oh, Tina, don't get upset. You don't have to worry about it now. The time when all this is going to happen is so far away. Let's just forget I even told you."

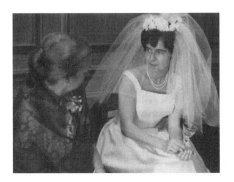
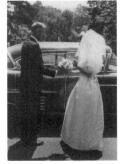

Hans:
"The time to start thinking about the last part of
my life is still so far away. You know I am just
starting up my new business. I'd be crazy to
move out of this house for another ten or fifteen
years, at least. I am too busy to think about
retiring out in the countryside!"

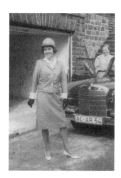 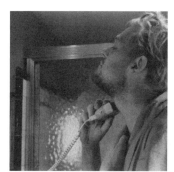 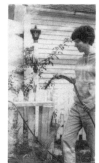

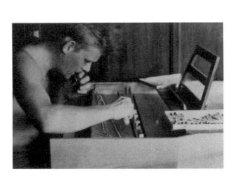

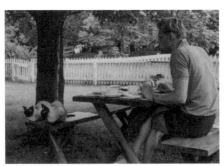

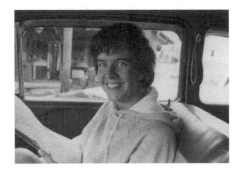

Contents

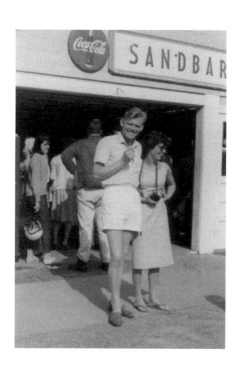

Introduction

How Things Turn Out

Parents encourage or discourage, praise or scold, remain silent or yell, and yet despite these influences, children grow up to have their own unique quirks and personality traits. In part, we become who we are to protect ourselves from the people we love who can hurt us. I didn't quite grow up the way my parents expected. But by their own admission, they didn't fulfill all their parents' expectations either. Neither did their parents . . . and so on.

My mother always wondered how she raised a daughter who enjoyed hugging so much. She never liked long embraces with anyone over the age of four. I could never get enough of them. I lived as a young adult in a very conservative rural area where physical affection was traditionally avoided, and I suffered severe withdrawal from lack of contact. I even took up martial arts as a hobby partially because it allowed me just to *touch* someone. Periodic sprains and fractures seemed a small price to pay.

It just goes to show that not everything turns out as planned. At least, that has been a central theme in my adult life. Nothing prepared me for the radical but methodical approach my mother took toward her own aging. Or *not* aging, which was actually her point. I'm not talking about plastic surgery to lift her chin or the daily consumption of a bowl of oat bran. She intended to implement a more aggressive strategy for dealing with the uncertainty of growing old. And I rebelled against her in an extraordinary battle of wills.

My father, on the other hand, always avoided setting a detailed agenda for his senior years. He lived in the moment, never looking far ahead, and we both anticipated his easy and pleasant retirement.

But a series of sudden, apocalyptic events derailed his dream and both our lives.

MY PARENTS EMIGRATED TO the United States from Germany in the late 1950s. They met here, and my brother and I were born in Toledo, Ohio. Approximately ten years after they married, they divorced. Both entered their sixties in relatively good health, except that my mother had chronic high blood pressure and my father had high cholesterol.

The true story I tell here (I have sometimes changed names of individuals and locations) focuses on my parents as they neared the ends of their lives—the time between 2003 and 2008. During these years my mother determinedly put in motion the plan she had hatched decades earlier, and I shouldered the burden of my father's rapidly deteriorating life.

Despite describing my parents in detail, this book is chiefly a narrative about me. I originally intended to tell *their* tales, from *their* perspectives. I did not get far with that, before having to interject fiction, assumption, repetition, and sheer fantasy into the mix. So instead I recount here, in my own voice, what I know best: myself, and how I reacted to experiences my parents and I shared.

Our family issues in many respects mirror those faced by most people. We had our measure of dysfunction; each of us carried some emotional baggage passed down from previous generations; we grieved deeply and loved as best we could; and we feared losing each other and losing the structure of life that bound us together. If you identify with some elements of this story, be kind to yourself as you read.

Sometimes we think we know how things are going to turn out—a drive to the grocery store, next year's vacation, the book lying on the bedside table. They all seem so predictable. And having a predictable ending can make the entire process more enjoyable, or at least more comforting.

But sometimes the process itself, not the foreseeable consequences, sets the tone, allows for change, and provides new opportunities for growth. My parents' final journeys were not easy, for them or for me. Yet each of us achieved a large measure of personal growth in the process, despite the suffering, and perhaps even because of it.

We all face permanent loss in our lives—loss of parents, loss of other relatives, loss of close friends. The process wrenches our souls, but it also reveals them. In this book I tell a personal story, but I believe the lessons are collective. When the time comes to deal with inevitable loss, solace and companionship may be found within these pages.

Chapter 1

The Phone Call

2007, 2001

In October 2007, I came home from an early-afternoon bike ride through the colorful Massachusetts foliage to find a solitary new message on our answering machine. The red light blinked insistently at even intervals, and while I had planned to run to the bathroom after removing my helmet and bike shoes, I decided I'd better listen to the recording. Standing in the kitchen next to the machine, I couldn't understand much of what the caller was saying, and I was tempted to delete the message as just another phone solicitation. I nevertheless pushed the repeat button and listened again: crackle, "I'm sorry," murmur, "your daddy," something incomprehensible, name of my father's nursing home, blah, blah, "very sad," something else incomprehensible, mumble, "call back."

Okay, I thought, *I don't need to get every word to understand this. They never call me. "I'm sorry . . . your daddy . . . very sad." I know what they're trying to tell me.* I scrambled to get my cell phone out of my pocket, then scrolled through the too-long contacts list. *My father, Hans, is dead.* I glanced up at the clock to remember the time. *One thirty-eight in the afternoon. But wait. Why didn't they call my cell phone after they realized no one was home?* Those were the nursing home's instructions: if something happened, they were to call me at home, then on my cell, then at work, then call Ron's cell. With four numbers, they were almost certain to be able to reach one of us.

Hans's nursing home was in Delaware, the state where he resided for most of his life. Until the beginning of 2007, Ron and I lived near Delaware as well. Then a change in my career brought us to Massachusetts. Rather than subject Hans to a grueling, disruptive move, the family chose to keep him near his friends and my brother. Nevertheless, I determined that the nursing home should always be able to reach me, because I had primary responsibility for his affairs.

I had emphasized the importance of having numerous ways to contact me because my father had specific orders on his chart: "Do not resuscitate. Do not hospitalize." Despite these directives, when he had been found unresponsive at five in the morning the previous year by a nurse at Lovering Nursing Home, she had called 911 first and me second. By the time I spoke with her, an ambulance was already transporting my father to the emergency room. After that incident, I learned my lesson. I taped a large sheet of paper to the front of Hans's chart. In all capitals it read, "DON'T CALL 911. CALL DAUGHTER." Then it listed my numbers.

I finally came to the middle of the alphabet on my phone and found the nursing home's listing. I pushed Send. As I waited for a connection, I felt strangely calm. *I hope he didn't suffer too much. But in any case his frustration and distress have ended.*

A woman with a strong Jamaican accent answered the telephone. I told her my name, that I was Hans's daughter, and that I had received a phone call from them. By the time I heard the first few words, "I'm so sorry to tell you that your father . . . ," I had finished her sentence in my mind: *is dead.* To my shock, she concluded instead, ". . . has been crying and screaming all morning. We thought that if you talked with him, you might be able to calm him down."

Not what I had anticipated. Not even close. "Oh. Right. Sure," I responded, fumbling for words. "I would be happy to talk with him."

"Good. We'll get him. Hold on."

I had only a moment to pull my thoughts back from the abyss into which they had mistakenly jumped. *It's* not *over.* And now I was standing in the kitchen really having to go to the bathroom—and instead waiting for the nursing home staff to wheel my father from his room to the nurses' station phone. *Why didn't I pee before I called?* But, of course, you don't think of that when you've just received a message seeming to indicate that your father has died. Before death, all your needs—physical, emotional, relational, financial—suddenly disappear into an arena far removed from daily life. After a while, it becomes difficult to make the effort to retrieve them.

For the previous two years, I'd been very good at shoving many of my needs under the rug out of concern for my father. Dangerously good. *After all, this is what a good daughter is expected to do.* Or so I thought.

My father cared for me his entire cognizant life, even when caring necessitated performing less than pleasurable duties. Though after their divorce my mother could be quick to enumerate Hans's faults, she always described him as an enthusiastic parent. For decades she even saved a copy of the letter Hans had written to family and friends the day after my birth, titled "The Report of a Proud Father." Therefore, I'm sure that during my childhood, along with cuddling and playing with me, Hans changed my diapers, cleaned up my vomit, and wiped my feverish brow. And I'm sure he did it with love for me in his heart.

WHEN MY PARENTS DIVORCED because of "irreconcilable differences," I was nine and my brother, Warner, was eight. My mother moved out of the house, which was uncommon at the time. Irmgard had initiated the separation; she had outgrown the marriage, so she was the one who left. Our parents gave Warner and me the choice of going with her or staying with Hans, and we made the most rational decision we could at the time: we asked, "Where will Speedy live?"

Speedy, the family cat, clearly favored my father. So Irmgard moved to an apartment complex three blocks away, and Speedy, Warner, and I continued to live in the large house with Hans.

Instead of alimony, our parents agreed to a one-time, lump-sum payout. Consequently, my father quickly found himself financially strapped, having borrowed money to pay my mother. All of a sudden, to our horror, and for no reason we could comprehend, my brother and I faced mealtimes with single frozen dinners split among the three of us, mountains of egg noodles or instant mashed potatoes, and foamy glasses of powdered milk. Used to our father's gourmet cooking with fresh ingredients and nightly variations on culinary themes, we rebelled vociferously against every cutback, but most especially against the frothy, tepid milk substitute. We hated the taste, the temperature, and the smell. We spat it out or refused to drink it, and eventually Hans acquiesced. After weeks of heated battle, we happily found the gallon jugs of fresh whole milk in the refrigerator once again. Our father had given in, a sign of his true love for us, we were certain.

The actual reason behind the sudden curb in spending remained unknown to us, as did the pain our constant complaining caused Hans. But we found out many years later that we had also been oblivious to his nightly pilgrimages to the kitchen. Close to midnight, moving quietly so as not to wake us, he would mix powdered milk with water, then rinse out the same plastic container that proclaimed in red letters, "Whole milk, vitamin D enriched," and funnel in the reconstituted milk, allowing the foam to settle overnight in the refrigerator. He fooled us every time.

I DIDN'T THINK OF what I did for Hans in the nursing home as reciprocating, doing for him just because he had done for me. I loved him, and I had firsthand knowledge that he did not shy away from putting aside his own needs and desires for the sake of his children's well-being.

Sometimes I held my breath out of a desire to avoid the reality of the moment, such as when I pulled his diapers down to help him pee. His penis could start to dribble before he bent his legs enough to sit on the raised toilet seat in the shared bathroom of his nursing home room. I would grab his organ and redirect the stream toward the toilet bowl, so that the urine didn't make too big a mess on the floor.

If I'm being honest, the entire procedure disquieted me. I know many children do much more for their elderly parents, but I would have been very content to go through my life without ever having had to touch my father's penis.

But sometimes I could not avoid it, because when my father had to go, he had to go *now*. Lovering was small and adequately staffed, but Hans didn't always give a lot of advance notice about his bodily functions, and he wasn't capable of much self-control. The feeling of urgency would overtake him suddenly, perhaps because he could no longer process the subtle early warning signs. I did not always have enough time to run down the hall to find a staff person to perform the duty I would rather have shirked. But I abhorred the alternative of letting him sit in wet diapers until someone could come around to change him. If he could tell me he had to empty his bladder, then he would realize his behind was not dry. Only my hang-ups stood in the way of his comfort. So I held my breath and tried to think of more pleasant things.

But caring for my father didn't feel the same as caring for a small child, although he was in many senses exactly that, and many of the routines were similar. Except he did not grow up—he grew down. He used to walk by himself, then he shuffled, then he moved along with a walker, and finally he was confined to a wheelchair. The scope of what served as his memory became ever more truncated, to the point where he lived almost exclusively from moment to moment. On the ubiquitous "activities of daily living" scale my father scored very low. He couldn't shave or bathe himself. Most days he could shovel food into his mouth, though it behooved his caregivers that he wore a bib. Still, he retained some of his old gestures, such as the way he put his huge hand up through my hair against the grain and ever so gently rubbed my scalp with his fingers; or the way his eyes sometimes gleamed with recognition of me. And his voice was the same—even if his words often followed a logic only he could comprehend.

"HI, HANS," I SAID into my cell phone when they brought him to the nurses' station and handed him the receiver. "It's . . ." But he interrupted. He knew me by the sound of my voice.

"Oh! Tina. How are you?" he choked out, his voice reverberating with emotion.

"I'm doing really well, Hans. How are you?" I responded, rather surprised that he had asked. He usually didn't. Quickly I added,

"How are you feeling?" because I learned he didn't always know how to respond to abstract questions such as how he was. A concrete question about his feelings derailed the conversation less often. The many possible answers regarding the state of his existence may have confused him. Or perhaps *how* he was linked too closely in his mind with similar questions having to do with *where* he was or *when* he was. The answers to these questions he did not know.

"Tina, I'm trying to figure out a . . . crossword puzzle," he said, "and I don't know the answers."

I knew with assurance that Hans was not solving a crossword puzzle. He hadn't read anything since his first major stroke. I had piled all manner of books and old magazines, even reading material from my childhood—illustrated editions of *The Cricket in Times Square* and *James and the Giant Peach*—on the desk in his room. But he lacked the initiative and the visual acuity to pick any of them up. Instead I responded to the emotional content of what he said: "It sounds like you're frustrated."

"Yes, I'm frustrated. I just can't figure it out. This crossword puzzle . . ." The thought trail ended abruptly for him. The subject shifted. "I was talking with Walter, and he said he was in the garden with you, but you were far away from him on the other side, and he couldn't speak with you. You didn't come over to talk with him. Maybe when he can speak with you, he can understand what's going on. Walter wants to wait to talk with you first. He doesn't want to talk with me, and you can't answer, either."

Walter was Hans's only brother, one year older, who still lived in Germany. Walter had probably called him recently. Being on the phone with me may have reminded Hans of this, or of being trapped in East Germany in his youth, or of any number of other past events. Having a conversation with Hans felt like being awakened suddenly in strange surroundings and thinking, "Where am I? What day is it? What am I doing here?" My mind would hurriedly grasp at the fragments of information in his sentences, trying to piece together the puzzle of his thoughts. I knew I could try to redirect the conversation, or I could continue in his world as best I could. This time I stuck with the concrete: "It's quite possible that Walter called you a few days ago."

"Yes, maybe I talked with Walter on the phone. But he won't tell me what's going on. He wants to speak with you, but you won't tell me either."

Nurses talking in the background interrupted us. They were speaking so loudly that for a while I thought they might have been talking to me. Then I realized they must have been having a conversation quite close by, not noticing my father on the phone. I asked Hans whether there were people around him. He replied that there were, but that he didn't know them.

In the seconds of silence I let pass, I tried to come up with an explanation of these people's presence to fit with the crossword-puzzle-speaking-with-Walter-and-me-in-the-garden scenario. I simply couldn't. *Well, then, why lie?* And so I launched into the truth: "Hans, those are nurses. You're in a nursing home. A while ago . . ." I hesitated and calculated. *Can it really be over two years now? Two thousand five, September thirteenth. Yes, that's over two years ago.* I sighed and told him the truth. "I can't believe it's been two years, but over two years ago, you had a massive hemorrhagic stroke. You were lying on the floor of your condo for more than three days before we found you. You were in the hospital for a while, but basically you've been in nursing facilities since. So the people around you are there to take care of you. They're part of the staff of the nursing home."

I paused, my heart beating faster, to see how he would react.

"They're nurses. Yes, I see. Well, that explains what they're doing here. But I don't remember any of that."

"Actually, that's my point exactly," I answered, astonished that he had not countered my story of his incapacitation with disbelief. Having started down this road of truth-telling, I saw no reason to stop. "Having no memory is part of your problem. You've had three strokes. Each one could have killed you, but you've survived. But your mind was affected, and you have no short-term memory anymore. Recently, you seem to be losing your long-term memory too.

So you just don't remember. But they are nurses. You'll just have to trust me."

Amazingly, Hans accepted this story without argument. Maybe he had already forgotten the beginning before I reached the end. In any case, he didn't protest. This contrasted dramatically with his rebelliousness during every part of his post-stroke life in the first year.

HANS'S CHANGES BEGAN IN early July 2005. That month, as part of a general downsizing in preparation for retirement, my father moved out of the house where he had lived for thirty years and into an empty condo I owned. Sometime during his move, he had the smallest of three eventual hemorrhagic strokes. Because the effect was not dramatic, no one noticed when or how the first one happened. Conceivably, it occurred in his sleep. Afterward, his eyes remained bright blue. He still combed his short blond hair to the left. He continued to cut an imposing figure with his broad-shouldered, narrow-waisted build. But appearances can be deceiving. Over the course of a few minutes or hours, my father ceased to be the Hans he had been for seventy-four years and the person my brother and I had known our entire lives.

I think the months from July to September must have been among the most miserable of Hans's existence. Vaguely sensing that something wasn't quite right, he angrily maintained that what wasn't right was other people's fault. Muddled thoughts plagued him, and his life slowly crumbled into disarray. But he attributed the changes to the incompetence of others. Something about his accusations didn't feel accurate, however, and this bothered him.

Hans became very unhappy. Yet he could not grasp his altered psychology, just as I did not appreciate that vagaries of synaptic connections and blood flow could modify a person's seemingly fundamental personality traits. Generally optimistic and outgoing, my father hardly ever remained ill tempered for long. Only after Hans was institutionalized that fall and I took over all his affairs did I discover just how much he had changed. At his local bank branch, he had screamed at the workers. Some were friendly acquaintances who had known him for decades, but he berated them for long wait times and "mistakes" they made with his account. Staff at the nearby drug and electronics stores avoided him, because he continually brought back items and yelled at them for selling him "defective" products. He made trips downtown to reprimand his financial advisor about the "deliberately incomprehensible" statements. He also harshly rebuked my brother and me for trivialities at regular intervals.

Had I been aware of the entire picture, I would have intervened. As it was, his anger baffled me, and I feared for our seemingly fast-disintegrating relationship. Chagrined, I didn't mention anything to anyone. Warner didn't talk about his problems with Hans to me, either.

In retrospect, I ignored mountain-sized clues that something was very wrong. My father had a doctorate from the Massachusetts Institute of Technology. Extremely bright, and mechanically as well as artistically inclined, he had nevertheless called me down to the condo twice to help him plug in the telephone. It turned out he had used the nonworking line of the two lines going into the building, both clearly labeled. Another time he called me because he couldn't figure out why his brand-new answering machine, returned three times already, still didn't function. He had forgotten he had a second answering machine plugged into an upstairs jack that was intercepting all his calls.

And why didn't I question his new obsession with his bowels? Even vivid monologues about his supposed lack of "regularity" failed to clue me in. Every day, according to him, his intestines were on the brink of suffering a fatal stoppage. Shortly before the next stroke, he had informed me with earnest urgency, "If I don't have a bowel movement by tomorrow, I'm going to call 911!"

I found myself making all kinds of excuses for his behaviors. I attributed his odd conduct to symptoms of a mild depression. I blamed his sadness and irritation on his having given up the house. After all, he planned to use the condo only as a way station before moving to a retirement community. He faced profound life transitions.

The last time I saw him alone before his second stroke, he had a pained expression on his face as he tried to sort out some of his thoughts. Sympathizing with his confusion, I cupped his head in my hands and said lovingly, "Hans, it must be horrible to be inside your brain right now."

"Tina," he responded as he looked despairingly into my eyes, "you have *no* idea."

In retrospect, I did not.

BACK ON THE PHONE with my father at the nursing home, I told him that the nurses would take care of him. I was not sure he believed me. So I tried to assuage his anxiety further. "Their job is to help you. If you want anything, you can just ask them. And I will talk with them and try to sort out some of the problems you are having. Just let me try to help, okay?"

"Okay," he responded with sincerity. "But I don't think you or anyone else can help me with this crossword puzzle. I have some of the answers but . . . the clues are not clear. I can't figure out what the clues mean. It's very cryptic."

And so we returned to the beginning. Feeling a bit confused by the conversation, I took a deep breath and tried to mirror his feelings back to him: "I can tell that it must be very frustrating. Not being able to figure out what you are doing is very difficult."

"Yes! I am very frustrated."

"I'm sure you are. I understand. Hans, just let me take care of it. I'll make sure someone helps you." I kept my words and voice calm. My biggest frustration was not being able to touch him, to look in his eyes or stroke his hand reassuringly. Through physical contact I achieved one of the strongest forms of connection I had with him. Although I knew staff treated him well at Lovering, I also knew few people had the time or inclination to give him long hugs or stroke his chest for a few minutes to help him relax. Having only a phone connection limited my ability to soothe him, although sometimes nothing I could do calmed him for long. This time, I thought I had succeeded. *Now, Tina, carefully maneuver the conversation toward a gentle ending, and you'll both feel better.*

"Hans, things are going to be okay. But you sound a little tired. Are you tired?"

"Yes, of course I'm tired. I've been working very hard to put all of the pieces together."

"I bet you *have* been working hard. Why don't you take a rest? You can tell the nurses that you want to go back to your room to take a nap."

"That's a good idea," he agreed, sighing as he did so.

He sounded so sweet. I felt extremely sorry that he felt trapped, both in his mind and in his physical life. But the practical side of me knew that getting him to put down the receiver sometimes presented difficulties. He didn't recognize many of the normal social clues that signal endings. This time all seemed to be going well. Wanting to finish on a positive note he might be able to remember for a few minutes, I said, "Okay, Hans. Just give the phone back to the nurses and I'll call you again soon."

"Okay."

And then, my mistake: "I love you."

"Oh . . . Tina!" he wailed despairingly. My father, who nine times out of ten had absolutely no reaction to "I love you" or even "Goodbye," under certain, unpredictable circumstances let the words touch the depth of his loneliness and desolation. Unfortunately, this turned out to be one of those times. All of a sudden, it was as though none of our conversation had even taken place. He sobbed, in gut-wrenching heaves. But through them he was also saying goodbye and letting go of the phone. I heard the crying become fainter as he put the receiver down on the counter. But it continued to echo loudly through my head.

The nurse who had initially called me picked up the handset. "He's still crying," she stated flatly, a touch of accusation in her voice.

No kidding, I wanted to respond. *You try and get him to calm down from three hundred miles away. I had him calm. I just blew it at the end. You can't feel worse than I do about it*. Again, I pushed my reaction aside and took a deep breath. "I know," I replied. "I would be happy to try again . . ."

She broke in eagerly, with obvious relief in her voice, "Now? Let me get . . ."

"No, no, not now. Later. Give him a few minutes, and if he's still crying, feel free to give me a call back. I'll be happy to try again. And I'll call my brother and encourage him to visit this weekend if he wasn't already planning to come down."

"Oh." I heard the palpable disappointment in the single syllable. I wondered what she intended to write in that day's progress note. *The resident was agitated and crying. Called his daughter and asked her to talk to him. But talking with her just made things worse.*

I hung up my cell phone thoughtfully. I recognized that by tomorrow Hans would remember none of this. I also knew that someday he might not even remember me.

As I finally headed toward the bathroom, I made a mental note to put "whole milk" on the shopping list. I suddenly felt a strong need to hold on to a bit of family tradition.

NOT THAT OUR FAMILY was particularly traditional. In the mid-1970s, most children of divorced parents lived with their mother. Warner and I were the only children we knew who lived with their father and a cat.

Despite the physical distance, my mother and I maintained a close relationship. Of course we had our disagreements, especially as I moved through my teenage years. Two people both holding tightly to the attitude, "I'm right and everyone else is crazy," easily ran into trouble. In general, though, our interactions were grounded in the mutual affection and respect we had for each other.

Yet Irmgard frequently pushed the two of us more and more toward mutual independence, toward what she considered a more equitable, self-reliant relationship. Sometimes I rebelled at what I perceived initially to be abandonment, only to realize after a period of acclimation that the new territory to which she had led us promised more enrichment, if only because it offered both of us more freedom. At first her request not to call her "Mom" anymore sounded harsh. I was in college at the time, enjoying a taste of adulthood, but I had no desire to cut all childhood ties. Still, after months of calling her, and then ultimately Hans, by their first names, I embraced the sense of equality this offered. And the woman I called Irmgard became more than a mother: she was my best friend.

In her retirement, Irmgard loved to scope out on foot the noteworthy areas of her adopted hometown, Wilmington, Delaware. Only when she declared a spot "delightful" would she share the experience with me. So it came to pass that she and I were walking on a sunny and mild Saturday morning in January 2001 along the downtown waterfront. We planned to visit the newly renovated and tenanted shops and restaurants she had previously investigated and to choose one of the cafés to have lunch in. Two women out to enjoy the winter sunshine: one small of stature but sure of stride, with dyed-blond hair and barely visible gray roots, the other taller and broad-shouldered, struggling to keep her long brown hair from blowing into her eyes.

But I do not remember the sparkling of the sun on the water, the café where we planned to eat, or the revitalized factory structures. Instead I remember the deep black of the pavement. It came zooming up toward my head to envelop me in darkness when I realized what my mother had just revealed.

I have frozen the moment in time. I can still see my foot raised in the air to step off the curb; can see it descending slowly. And then I lost my footing—the instant I realized my sixty-six-year-old mother had decided to kill herself before she turned seventy.

Chapter 2

The Birthday Party

2001

My conversation with Irmgard began innocently enough. My father's seventieth birthday was rapidly approaching. As the master planner of the family, I appointed myself in charge of the festivities. Months earlier, I asked my father if he would like a large party, remembering his last milestone birthday, the big five-oh. I was fifteen then and had teased him by commenting, "You're so old!" He replied seriously, "Tina, you only have two choices in life: you get older or you die. Of the two, I prefer getting older." My father still believed this. He enthusiastically supported the idea of a party celebrating his seven decades, especially when I insisted he, for once, stay out of the kitchen and actually enjoy his own event.

As my mother and I walked in the sunshine, enjoying the view of the river, I regaled her with plans for the occasion. Although she and Hans had been divorced almost thirty years, under most circumstances she could still bring herself to be only icily civil about "your father." Sometimes she barely mustered even that much self-control. After years of listening to claims that Hans's indolence caused his chronic back problems, his unwise decisions resulted in his financial worries, and even the Japanese beetle invasion of his garden was somehow the product of a festering character defect, I laid down a firm rule: Don't criticize Hans to me—I'm not taking sides. From that point on she managed to keep most of her complaints about Hans to herself.

Hoping she would not find the topic of Hans's birthday too objectionable, I continued. "I've ordered vegetarian sushi," I enthused, as my longer legs worked hard to keep up with her always energetic though short stride. "Hans loves sushi, but I didn't want to risk the fish going bad. And I'm investigating where to get some other types of food—maybe Thai?"

"How many people are coming?"

"I think there could be about fifty, if everyone shows up. It's so nice that they're making the effort to come. Much better to have this kind of event when everyone is still healthy."

"Tina, you know my philosophy about that," Irmgard chuckled. "I went to see my brother in Germany after his heart attack, remember? All my relatives were so surprised I came all that way when he wasn't even dead! And then I told them they shouldn't expect me to go to his funeral. That shocked them, of course." She smiled and glanced up at me impishly.

IRMGARD DID NOT SHY away from shocking people. She maintained she had lived an obedient and docile youth, and I had no reason to doubt her. But I always harbored a suspicion that as she aged, she increasingly went out of her way to appear eccentric, perhaps because she had simply tired of the commonplace. Sometimes the twinkle in her eye betrayed the mischievous intent behind an ostensibly innocent remark.

Yet in describing my mother's personality, I would never use the word mischievous. Instead, I would call her most striking quality "strength of character"—or I would call it stubbornness; passionately embraced beliefs, or an inability to see another point of view; devotion to long-held principles, or cold rationality. However expressed, it also represented her Achilles' heel.

As an example, Irmgard left Germany in the 1950s, in her midtwenties. After marrying my father, she remained in the United States and saw her German relations infrequently. Yet despite the passage of decades, her impression of her relatives fixedly endured, frozen at the point when she had left the country. To my mother, one brother was forever a teenage delinquent, another a quiet preadolescent. Each family member perpetually played the same role.

As everyone aged, Irmgard rationalized present-day events to fit past personalities. Once, when she and I visited Germany together, she overheard her sixty-year-old, formerly aberrant and antisocial brother offer to carry his wife's heavy suitcase. Irmgard commented loudly and embarrassingly to him and the entire hotel lobby, "Wow, he's never done anything like that before! He's acting like a gentleman. This must be a once-in-a-lifetime event!" That her brother had matured in the forty intervening years did not occur to her. Change simply did not fit her version of the family's dynamics.

Irmgard's unwillingness to alter her beliefs earned her both loyal friends and bitter enemies. My mother's allies occupied a privileged position. She declined to let anyone but a select few fully into her heart, and as long as no rift occurred, she staunchly supported those she loved and earned their trust in return. But enemies of my mother disappeared down the well of time. Capable of ignoring the passage of years, she could also cut someone suddenly and completely out of her life. I saw it happen in as little as a day and for as little as a misspoken word.

Nevertheless, for much of my early life with her, I felt enveloped in a cocoon of affection. If I looked pretty to myself, I looked "stunning" to her. If I did well in school, I was a genius. If I painted a mediocre woodland scene, she had it professionally framed and hung it proudly on her wall, crooked trees and all. When I walked around her condominium, even decades later, seeing my brother's kindergarten clay figure, my certificate of special achievement in ninth-grade French, a small wooden chest I built in shop class, and a wall hanging my brother stitched for her at summer camp—all still prominently displayed—did not surprise me.

One afternoon when I was in first grade and Warner in kindergarten, we were not there to meet our mother outside school at the appointed pickup time. After searching the school building, Irmgard finally spied us sitting on the floor of the library. Neither of us noticed her enter the room. Intent on the activity at hand, we bent over our small feet, oblivious to all but our shoelaces. As teacher, I patiently recited, "Over, under, around, and through," moving my hands in time with my words. Warner, as student, concentrated intently on my actions and tried to mimic them with his own laces. He failed repeatedly. Over, under, around, and through, again and again, until finally, in one fluid motion, Warner tied his laces and jumped up in excitement. Only then did we notice our mother looking at us, beaming with joy at our mutual success. It had taken us almost an hour. And she had watched us in silence the entire time.

Even as an adult, I never doubted that my mother was my strongest and most loyal fan, the only person on earth with the self-proclaimed hobby of "Tina-watching."

We walked along the Wilmington riverbank that day, and Irmgard pointed out names of companies that had moved into the renovated buildings. I babbled on about my father's party. "You should see the paper I found for the invitations. It has colorful balloons all around the edges."

"That sounds nice, Tina."

Suddenly, a thought struck me. I remember wondering at the time why it hadn't occurred to me sooner. I slowed my pace. "Look, Im," I said, calling her by my personal nickname for her. "I know you don't like parties in general, but don't you think it could be fun to celebrate *your* seventieth birthday like this, too?"

My mother didn't answer, instead turning the corners of her mouth upward in a secret smile.

I took this as my cue to sell her on the positive possibilities. "I know it's still four years away. But it would be fun to think about. We could invite a lot of your friends, even people in Germany. Wouldn't it be great to see them? It would be in keeping with the whole idea you had when you visited your sick brother that time, wouldn't it? See them while you're still healthy, instead of having them come to your funeral?"

My mother began to look slightly uncomfortable. I interpreted her discomfort as caving in under the power of my argument. I continued: "We could have it be anything you want. We wouldn't have to have decorations; we wouldn't even have to advertise the birthday

aspect. We could just make it an occasion to get everyone together."
I paused.

She finally spoke. "Tina, you know it's hard for me to say no to you, but I don't like the idea. Have a good time planning Hans's party. I don't need one."

I couldn't understand what she disliked. I pressed her.

"But why don't you like it? I could make it completely unstressful for you. You could be in control of everything, so it would be just what you want . . ."

"Okay, Tina," she suddenly relented, her voice lowering to almost a whisper. "Why don't we just say that you're going to have this party for me when I turn seventy? You just do it any way you want. Invite anyone you like."

Great! I thought, and then halted before reacting. *Wait . . . that was too easy. And why doesn't she care about how it's done?* For a few moments, a cacophony of connecting synapses overwhelmed me. Then, clear as a single note, a realization emerged from the dissonance: My mother had no interest in the party and would let me plan it any way I wanted, because she had no intention of being around.

THIS WASN'T EXACTLY NEWS to me. For over a decade I had been living with abstract knowledge of my mother's plans.

When she had been in her mid-fifties, Irmgard had decided she would cut her life short before she reached old age. I was then in my twenties. And she told me all about it.

"Tina, it's my life, and I can do what I want. But I'm also doing this for you. I don't want to burden you or Warner with having to take care of me when I can't care for myself any longer. You won't want to have to change my diapers or have me look at you and not know who you are."

"But Im, . . ."

"No, wait. Let me finish. I also want to leave you a little money. I don't have much, but I don't want to use it all up on some big hospital or nursing home bill. And it's also because I have always been scared of death. But now that I've decided I'm not going to leave that final event to chance, I feel much better. I can be in control of it, and this gives me a kind of inner peace nothing else can."

"Wait. Please listen to me. I don't want you to do it!"

"Oh, Tina, don't get upset. You don't have to worry about it now. The time when all this is going to happen is so far away. Let's just forget I even told you."

My mother had told me she was going to kill herself and I was supposed to forget about it? How could I? Rationally, I tried to understand her reasons. But as a young adult, I couldn't begin to imagine what taking care of an ailing parent would involve. Changing her diapers? Watching her lose her mind? *Not easy*, I thought. But having her die? *No way!*

I never for a moment wanted her to follow through with her plan. I told her repeatedly in subsequent conversations I hated the idea of life without her. I certainly didn't want her to end her life to protect *me* from her old age. I wanted her with me as long as possible. It didn't matter to me what shape she was in.

Consistently, she brushed my arguments aside. "It's so many years away, Tina. It's not even worth discussing now."

From the moment of that first conversation, I lived with the sword of Damocles hanging over my head. I told myself she was correct, that these events were too far in the future to overshadow my life in the present. I told myself she might change her mind. I told myself all these things. I didn't convince myself of any of them.

As with my father's lighthearted declaration about old age, "Grow older or die," with my mother I also faced only two choices: accept her wishes or be shut out. I could rail against them, but those who knew Irmgard best knew the futility of arguing with her most deeply held convictions. And they understood that she would penalize those who opposed her with exile.

IRMGARD POSSESSED AN EXCEEDINGLY strong desire to remain in control of her own faculties, partially because she appreciated the precariousness of a person's health in general and her own in particular.

Since my birth, she had suffered from high blood pressure. Initially untreated, it led to her having a stroke in 1972. She was just thirty-eight, and I was in second grade.

At the time, Warner and I attended school in a suburb of Toledo. Every morning my mother drove us there, a normal occurrence for most of the student body. But Irmgard did not chauffeur us to the main entrance like the other mothers. Instead, rain or shine, wind or snow, she stopped at the edge of an unused lot that bordered the school's playing fields and led to a ravine. Every day my brother and I walked the path leading into the tall grass. We regarded it as a long, arduous trek full of mystery and fraught with potential danger. As we approached the deep ravine, our hearts beat faster. The adventure thrilled us—the descent into a world below eye level, its damp coolness, its potentially shoe-snatching clay. The banks towered over our heads, engulfing us for fifty feet until we clambered gratefully up the muddy edge on the other side. Breathing more easily, we ran the remaining yards across the shorn grass to the front doors of the school. Always during this journey, Warner and I turned back periodically to wave at my mother. A reassuring presence, guarding our passage with enthusiastic waves back to us, she remained by her car, watching until we entered the building.

Now as an adult I understand that the walks originated in her upbringing, with the German belief in the importance of daily physical exercise. Back then I thought Warner and I could not get to school any other way. The other children arrived by car. This family walked. A car luxuriously appeared at the school doors only for our ride home.

Yet one afternoon my father, not my mother, sat in the parking lot outside school, waiting to pick us up. "Get in," he told us through the open window.

"Where's Mom?" Warner and I asked him simultaneously.

"Just get in," he repeated. "I'll explain on the way."

The sudden disappearance of our normal routine disturbed us, and we sat taciturnly in the back of the station wagon as our father wound his way among the cars exiting the school's driveway. After he had merged onto the main road, he kept his explanation short. "Your mother's in the hospital, and we're going to see her now."

So I assume Irmgard's stroke must have happened sometime during the day. As children, we did not ask how Irmgard contacted my father at work, what symptoms she felt, and who transported her to the hospital. For us, Mom was gone, and we had no idea where she was. Hospital meant about as much to us as "Kathmandu." We only understood she wasn't at home, and things were no longer the same. When we saw her, she sat in a white bed, in a room with white walls and a white floor. She wore a white gown. Lots of white—that impressed us.

I dutifully repeated the hospital visitation story to my teachers at school the next morning, after having memorized the words "My mother had a stroke." I had also mastered a second phrase: "blood pressure." As the days passed, my teachers never ceased to be interested in this puzzling blood pressure phenomenon. Every day they asked, and every day I informed them of seemingly random digits my father had impressed upon me in the morning, such as "two hundred over one hundred thirty." Depending on which numbers I repeated and in which order, their faces contorted with concern or relaxed into relief. I remember my heart racing, fearing I had said the wrong numbers or inverted the sequence. The figures ranged into integers far outside my second-grade-math comfort zone.

Eventually my mother returned home, and the experience faded in the usual rush of childhood. It became ancient history—somehow relevant but not of immediate concern. Then ten years later, in 1982, I visited Germany for part of the summer after my junior year in high school. I stayed with Irmgard's brother, and one afternoon he called me to the phone.

"Tina, don't be afraid," my mother began. "I have to tell you something, but don't worry. Everything is fine now. I'm in a hospital in Maine. Two weeks ago, while I was here on vacation, I had a heart attack. I'm better now. Please believe me. Everything is okay."

Certainly, I did not want to hear this kind of news while separated from my mother by an ocean. But a later angiogram revealed that only one-sixth of her heart had ceased to function, and she faced no other lasting consequences. Her life returned to normal, as did mine. Eventually that event, too, faded into the past.

In the decades after her heart attack, however, my mother gradually instituted some extreme behavior changes aimed at improving her health. She named her new state "terminally healthy." By her mid-sixties, she had embraced vegetarianism and ate mostly uncooked vegetables and fruit. She completely stopped drinking alcohol and caffeine. She avoided fat and sugar. She exercised religiously, power walking outside at least an hour every day, in icy conditions retreating to her treadmill.

Despite these alterations, her blood pressure remained high. Still, she refused to take medications. She insisted the radical adjustments to her lifestyle should be sufficient. Then in 1997, after a brief hospitalization with a serious bout of pneumonia, she changed her views. She realized a premature stroke before her final plan could be put into effect would ruin well-thought-out preparations. From then on, she took daily blood pressure medication, and her blood pressure relaxed to normal levels.

BACK AT THE WATERFRONT I recovered from my stumble. I turned to my mother, shivering slightly with a foreboding chill. "Wait. What you're actually telling me is that you have no intention of being around for your seventieth birthday. You're going to kill yourself before then, right?"

She tried to laugh it off. It was a fake laugh, and we both knew it.

"Right? I'm right, aren't I?" I said, my voice quavering with intermingled anger, shock, and sadness.

I absorbed the enormous ramifications of her statement, and my stomach clenched as though she had struck me. I knew my mother. When she made up her mind to do something, not even her beloved children could stop her.

"Tina, I didn't want to tell you."

"If you didn't want to tell me, why did you say it just now?"

"I didn't mean to. You were pushing so hard. I didn't know what to say."

I scowled at her, my face flushed with outrage and grief. "I don't believe you. If you hadn't wanted me to know, you wouldn't have said anything. Or you would have lied." I paused.

This new piece of information overwhelmed me, but I had to know more. "So, now you've told me. What's your plan? When are you going to do it?"

Chapter 3

Origins
2008

When my brother and I were little we fought like . . . well, like brothers and sisters. Separated in age by just one year and twenty-one days, we felt all the rivalry of fraternal twins but not much of the camaraderie.

Looking back at our earlier years, I wonder how much of our constant antagonism reflected our parents' continual battles. Each entrenched in a viewpoint and unwilling to empathize with the other, our parents provided little constructive relationship role modeling. Irmgard and Hans both later told me about their happy first years together. But I personally never experienced them as a loving couple. By the time I could retain memories, their relationship had already soured. The divorce ended most of the yelling, but hard feelings remained. And for many years, Warner and I continued to act out the drama our parents had taught us.

One day when we were nine and ten, I kicked a hole in Warner's solid-wood bedroom door. As we did many afternoons, we assumed our usual fighting positions. I twisted his doorknob from the outside and shoved with both hands to get in. He jammed his foot up against the bottom and leaned into it with all his weight to keep it shut. I finally vented my frustration by giving a few mighty kicks to the lower panel.

Our rage momentarily evaporated as the panel splintered and we saw my sneaker-clad foot suddenly sticking through what we had both taken to be an unyielding barrier. Shortly, our shock reconfigured itself into righteous indignation. We heard the familiar clanking of my father's diesel station wagon enter the driveway. He had returned from work. We shoved each other on our way down the carpeted stairs, rounded the sharp bottom corner by the front door, and raced along the hallway toward the kitchen in the back of the house. Breathless and still jostling, we assailed my father the second he stepped through the back door. Each of us hoped to convince him of our "helpless victim" status in the crime. Worn out from a long day at the lab and gearing himself up to cook dinner, he couldn't even put down his overcoat before we assaulted him with our divergent accounts of the preceding half hour.

"Dad, Warner yelled at me for no reason and slammed his door in my face," I began.

Not wanting to be out-shouted by his older and taller sister, Warner broke into a full yell: "Dad, Tina came into my room even though I told her not to, and then she took my Sherlock Holmes book without asking. When I tried to get it back . . ."

Wearily used to these homecomings, my father immediately retreated without a word to his upstairs bedroom to smoke his pipe and wait things out. We could smell the scent of Captain Black tobacco wafting from under his door. He refused to emerge and prepare dinner until we'd calmed down. Hunger quickly prevailed over anger this time, but Warner and I experienced only fleeting intervals of peace.

With the adults off in their respective base camps, we children fought the ongoing war of our family in the trenches. Although we have mellowed with age and now find many things to agree on, Warner and I have carried our scars far into adulthood. Despite this, we have also learned to communicate and to see each other's perspective.

My parents never discovered how to do that with each other.

IRMGARD AND HANS BOTH grew up in Germany in the 1930s and '40s. They both experienced the Second World War as young teenagers. They both came to the United States in the late 1950s to escape their pasts and create new identities. And by chance, they both ended up at M.I.T., where they met, my mother a lab technician and my father a graduate student.

After the divorce, those were the only parallels in their lives—except for some unusual and amusing similarities I discovered over time. They each vacationed in Japan, years apart, long after their divorce. They never spoke about their visit to each other, and yet they came home with the same souvenirs. "What's Hans's soy sauce container doing in your kitchen?" I once asked my mother with surprise.

"What are you talking about?" she responded, insulted. "That's *my* container."

"Well, there's another one exactly like it over in Hans's dining room," I replied. *Not only that, but the same wall hanging*, I thought it best not to add.

Then there was the time we all went to a protest march together. The old 1960s feeling of dissent in the air had been strong enough to get my parents to ride up to Philadelphia in the same car with me and my first husband. As I stomped down Broad Street in the crowd of demonstrators, warmly clad in layers of winter gear, my husband nudged me in the ribs with his elbow and leaned over to whisper in my ear, laughing, "Check out your parents' shoes and socks." I looked and saw four leather hiking boots and four woolen socks, identical down to the blue trim on the boots and the gray-and-maroon color of the stockings. So I know for sure my parents had at least one other thing in common: their aesthetic sense. Add to that their love for their children, and I can remember nothing else.

What ill will existed before their divorce they only exacerbated in its aftermath. Separated, neither of them worked at establishing anything but a tenuous truce. Recently, I found a single interoffice memo encased in a clear plastic sleeve that my father had kept in his files through the decades. I imagine he preserved it because it expressed something about the way he and my mother interacted. My parents worked at the same company, and they found it less provocative to use the company's mail system than to talk on the telephone. A conversation could easily escalate to yelling.

The note read:

Hans, July 31: I will be on a business trip to Chicago the
week of Aug. 17, Monday through Friday. Are you
interested in having Warner and Tina stay with you?
Irmgard, August 2: I am ALWAYS interested. It just doesn't
work out sometimes, or W & T are not interested.
Hans, August 4: Okay. Does it work out this time?
Irmgard, August 6: *Yes.*

How typical, my father must have thought. *Six days to get a straight
answer out of her!* Certainly, my mother's passive-aggression dominated this particular exchange, but I am sure my father had his
moments too. How could a relationship so rife with deliberate mis-
understanding end in anything but disaster?

How, somewhere long before, could these two people have been
madly in love?

ON A WEEKEND IN 2008, Ron was away at a conference and I went
on a cleaning rampage in our basement. I have to be in a special
state of mind to do more than everyday cleaning. So when the urge
to purge hits me, I make the time for it, knowing I will get rid of
things I would otherwise hold on to. That weekend, with Ron unable to tell me, "Don't throw that away!" I decided to spend a few
hours going through my parents' things, which I had carried with
me, without much inspection, from Pennsylvania to Massachusetts.

Stacks of solid-brown cardboard banker's boxes, piled six or
seven high, lined the back wall of the large downstairs room. I
switched on the rows of fluorescent ceiling lights. With everything
lit up like a football stadium, I decided to work my way from one
end to the other, starting with the boxes of my father's things and
ending with my mother's. I brushed away a fluffy ball of pink insula-
tion from the top box on the far left side. *How did the cat manage to
climb up here and rip that out of the ceiling?* I wanted to downsize,
eliminate the junk, and keep only what was still useful.

I had no idea that through this planned culling of possessions I would unearth enticing information about two then-young people I had never known.

What I imagined as a few hours of hard labor and easy decision making metamorphosed into a rhythmic routine that slowly revealed a puzzle. I carried a box from its place next to the wall, then sorted the objects into "junk," "shred," "keep," or "look at later." In the end, the last pile glued me to my work long after morning had turned into late afternoon. When the junk bags were tied shut and ready for the trash, I concentrated on the tantalizing bits and pieces I had come across. Set out in front of me on the floor, three boxes spilled out their contents: folders I had forgotten about, a photo album I'd never seen before, and stacks of papers and notebooks whose existence I had not known of. They beckoned with the appeal of a bestselling mystery on a bookstore shelf.

For very different reasons, neither my mother nor father preserved much information about their pasts. My mother moved frequently. For almost two decades she tried to outrun the conversion of one apartment building after another into condominiums. Although after relocating from Ohio she never lived outside Wilmington, she stubbornly resisted immobility being forced on her. Before she finally settled down, she had changed apartments six times, and with each move the number of her possessions diminished. She became more and more of a self-defined minimalist, rejoicing in her ability to live with less. Often she threw or gave away items related to her past: damask tablecloths, tea sets, sewing patterns, old diaries, photos.

In the year before her planned death she became even more extreme, condensing all her remaining loose photos into one small, clearly labeled and chronological album. She read once more and then discarded old letters. She gave away most of her books. She donated her clothing. I would have few sentimental objects to contend with after she was gone, she informed me. But what I discovered in my basement led me to believe she had been less detached from her past than she wanted to appear.

In contrast, my father hoarded sentimentally. For over thirty years in his three-story house, he accumulated all manner of possessions in the basement, in closets, in the attic, and in drawers. Then, as he prepared to move out of his home, he gradually brought order to some of the chaos, battling emotionally against the rush of memories. Working slowly, he painstakingly labeled things: "stay" or "go to condo." He also arranged for a professional service to clean out his house after he had moved, to remove everything he left.

Then he had his first stroke. The resulting addling of his brain prevented him from making rational decisions. As a consequence, a relatively large number of his prized possessions remained in the house instead of traveling with him. The cleaning service subsequently disposed of them at auction, thrift store, or landfill. Nevertheless, whether by luck or by decision, some photos and papers survived.

I found in my basement materials from my parents' magical years, the time after their emigration to the United States and before my birth. My father was movie-star handsome: six foot two, with thick, wavy blond hair and a square, well-proportioned face. He had a relaxed smile and shining blue eyes. In photos his large hands toy with cigarettes, pipes, and books. My mother, not quite equaling my father in good looks, capitalized on her thin figure, her dark hair and blue eyes, and her clear, earnest expression. She posed for photos, her head frequently sporting a late-1950s hat, with one leg before the other to accentuate her shapely calves.

At one time they may have possessed much more. But the things I found in those slightly musty boxes gave me a glimpse into a past I could never have imagined.

Chapter 4

A Long Road

1950s, 2008

My father's second life began on March 20, 1953, the day he fled East Germany for the West. A few days prior, he and his brother, Walter, received a short and innocuous phone call from their father. It ended with, "I'll see you at the Schreiners' on the twentieth," the code words their family had agreed on. That single sentence signaled the time to leave the East. The Schreiners lived in West Berlin, and everyone in the family headed there singly or in pairs, by different routes, so as not to arouse suspicion.

At the time, my father and Walter were both studying at the Mining Academy in Freiberg (not to be confused with Freiburg, the West German city). Escaping necessitated that they leave almost all their belongings behind. They packed one small, inconspicuous suitcase each and donned a number of layers of clothing. They then boarded a train to East Berlin. There, they entered a subway station and bought tickets for a stop within the West Berlin city limits. In those Cold War days, Berlin stood divided, but the wall had not yet been erected. The subway system still ran its old route throughout the city, heedless of international borders and no-man zones. To escape, one simply had to get on a subway car in the East and get off in the West. Only this method was neither simple nor safe. Commuters and shoppers crowded the cars, but so did East German police. If you looked suspicious, you could be pulled aside. If they found your luggage packed tightly with photos, money, or clothing, you would be interrogated, imprisoned, or worse. My father never spoke with me about that subway ride, but, having just turned twenty-two, he was probably terrified.

Luck was with the family members that day. They all eluded capture, met in West Berlin, and announced themselves at one of the refugee centers, where hundreds like them arrived daily. Good fortune had not always followed the family, however.

My father was born in 1931 and grew up in Hohenleipisch, a hamlet about sixty miles south of Berlin. My paternal grandfather owned a factory that made clay flowerpots and prided himself on being the big fish in this tiny village pond. In photos this third-generation potter is tall but slightly pudgy, with thinning hair, an approachable smile, and thick, dark-rimmed glasses. In addition to running the factory, the family also grew vegetables and fruit and maintained housing for some factory workers.

My grandfather groomed Walter, the older son, to take over the family business. Consequently somewhat ignored by his father, Hans gravitated toward his mother, spending much of his time in the kitchen. She cooked, ran the household, and served as the bookkeeper for the factory. And she doted on Hans, her baby.

Then came the war. Numerous times Russian and German troops passed through the area, using the citizenry to avenge their sense of nationalism. Russian soldiers raped German women who failed to conceal themselves behind wardrobes or in barn stalls. In retaliation, German soldiers shot Russian immigrant workers, leaving them for German youth, including my father, to bury. Both sides in turn burned entire sections of the village to the ground. My father rarely spoke of the war, but once he told me of being forced to climb a tall telephone pole to watch for approaching Russian soldiers. He perched precariously at the top for hours, as petrified of falling as he was of seeing the olive uniforms marching across the countryside.

Almost the entire family survived the war, even though in the final months Walter, then age fifteen, was conscripted and trained to drive a tank. Only my grandmother did not live to witness peace. Tragically, she died in 1943 of an ectopic pregnancy, one day after my father's thirteenth birthday.

My grandfather knew the signs; doctors had operated on his wife for the same condition before. When my grandmother started to experience pain and bleeding, my grandfather called for the single town ambulance to take her to the hospital several miles away. But during the war the ambulance was rigged to run on the only fuel readily available to civilians—wood. Spewing soot, it arrived, but after the attendants loaded my grandmother, the driver could not restart the engine. The family car had been commandeered by the army, so my desperate grandfather telephoned the German garrison stationed in town. The officer coldly informed him that no matter what the situation, military vehicles could only be used to transport military personnel. Eventually, the ambulance started. But by the time my grandmother arrived at the hospital, she had lost a great deal of blood. After an unsuccessful surgery, she slowly lost the feeling in her limbs. She died within a week.

Her death devastated my father. Even sixty years later, retelling this story brought tears to his eyes. As a young adult, the emptiness he felt from losing his mother eventually fueled a search for opportunities to create a new life. While his father and brother suffered emotionally from their loss of status after fleeing East Germany, Hans reveled in the new opportunities the West afforded and the chance to leave sad memories behind. Several years after their initial escape, the family was beguiled by the lies of the East German government. If they returned, they were told, there would be no reprisals and all property and status would be restored. But my father remained adamant. He had no ties there. He knew his future lay elsewhere and remained in West Germany alone.

After his family returned to Hohenleipisch, Hans widened his horizons even further. His heart still drawn to the family pottery tradition, he earned his master's degree in ceramics and worked for a company based in West Berlin. But he wanted more, something new. He went to the U.S. consulate and obtained a record of all American graduate schools offering PhDs in ceramics. The document ranked the schools from the most prestigious on down. To him, it was just a list. As soon as he received an acceptance letter, he stopped applying. That he had been admitted into one of the top schools came as a complete surprise to him. He often recounted, "On board the ship to the United States, I was taken aback by people's reactions when I mentioned M.I.T. Their eyes would widen in amazement and the conversation would suddenly stop. I thought M.I.T. must be a horrible place, because everyone seemed to react so negatively." In reality, the mental picture of a slightly impoverished-looking, poor-English-speaking, East German refugee attending such a renowned institution must have bewildered the seafaring Americans.

Oblivious to the demands of what lay ahead, my father arrived in New York Harbor on the SS *America* with all his possessions in one suitcase and one trunk. It was 1959, fourteen years after the war had ended. He was twenty-eight.

By 1958, MY MOTHER had already spent several years training as a metallographer at the Max Planck Institute in Düsseldorf, West Germany. Every weekend she commuted back to her small hometown, Altena, in North Rhine–Westphalia. The houses there nestled along both sides of a steep river valley, and as the train wound a sooty trail along the edge of the waterway, she hatched her liberation plans.

Born in 1934, my mother was the oldest of five children. She and two brothers were born before the war, and two more brothers came after. Her father ran a steel drawing factory that made wire for industrial use. In the home, he maintained tight discipline, enforced along the biblical lines cautioning against sparing the rod. In photos he appears austere, with thinning hair slicked back from his high forehead, thin lips pressed together tightly, and glinting eyes. My grandmother took care of the household and, according to my mother, dreamed secretly of her youth, when she had lived in a big city and danced through the night. In the pictures taken during her unfulfilling marriage, however, my grandmother also looks severe: her long hair tied up in a matronly bun, her clothing muted in color and conservative in cut, and her face reflecting the stifling atmosphere in which she lived.

Despite her parents' unhappy marriage, my mother had a privileged youth. The family was comparatively well-off. Her father nevertheless insisted on extreme frugality, in order that his children "not grow up spoiled." Still, when the Allies dropped bombs on the industrial area around Altena, my grandparents could afford to send my mother and her two brothers to live with relatives in the countryside, where they frolicked without school or adults to supervise them. Later, after British occupation forces commandeered the family home as officers' garrisons, everyone retreated to live in my grandfather's company offices. Other families were forced to flee to refugee shelters or relatives' living rooms.

As was customary, my grandfather prepared the oldest son in the family to take over the family business. The second-oldest son rebelled against his father's strict discipline and neglect. Becoming the family delinquent, he was sent off to boarding school. Having her father's watchful eye often turned elsewhere relieved my mother of the pressure to achieve. After the war, she cheerfully participated in raising her two youngest brothers, whom she adored. But my grandfather's discipline isolated her from her peers.

From the outside one can only look for clues about the darkness of life under my grandfather's stern rule. My mother's need for absolute control did not arise from blissful formative years. Although in her early youth Irmgard may have been the favorite child, she also warned me of her father's fickleness. When I went to visit my grandparents' home for summer vacation, she cautioned repeatedly, "Don't think your grandfather's going to love you forever. He loves you only until you start to have your own ideas. Then it gets nasty." She hated her father well into her adulthood, for reasons she never revealed. Over what exactly she and her father had clashed, I don't know. I do know that life in Altena reverberated with disturbing undertones.

My grandmother endured my grandfather's philandering, firing housemaid after housemaid as the truth emerged about his sexual liaisons with them. But she didn't suffer in silence. She threatened suicide daily, terrorizing my youngest uncle by warning him as he left for school that he would probably come home to find her body swinging from a rope in the attic. Now accomplished men in their sixties and seventies with grandchildren of their own, some of my uncles still have regular nightmares about their parents and their childhood home.

The older my mother grew, the stronger became her desire to escape from her stifling and stunting family life. Away from the dark valley, away from the rules and the bitterness, away from the endless melodrama of her parents' lives, my mother believed she could reach her own unique potential. Her first escape was to Düsseldorf to begin metallography training. Her second was to the United States.

My mother's practicum in Düsseldorf would end in the spring of 1958. In mid-1957 she began pulling strings to find a position in a university lab across the Atlantic. The letters and résumés she preserved document a convoluted series of connections, eventually landing her at the feet of one Nicholas Grant in the Department of Metallurgy at M.I.T. A highly intelligent and productive new full professor, said by his colleagues to be colorful and warm, Professor Grant must have seemed a welcome change from her father. He offered my mother a yearlong visa commitment in exchange for help with some of his research on metallic alloys.

With grudging approval from her parents for a temporary stay, my mother left West Germany. Early in the morning of October 8, 1958, two days before her twenty-fourth birthday, she disembarked from the SS *Statendam* in New York Harbor.

MY PARENTS ARRIVED IN the United States approximately nine months apart. It would be another three years before Hans invited Irmgard over for dinner at his apartment on Beacon Street in Brookline, Massachusetts, just outside Cambridge.

In the meantime, each separately adapted to life in the States. My father lived for a few months in a rented room but soon moved into a Blanche Street apartment with two roommates from China. The international atmosphere of the greater Boston area, the university, and his own living quarters energized him. Instead of balking at the creations his friends concocted in their tiny, shared kitchen, my father eagerly took part in cooking them. ("Get out the chopsticks! We're having Chinese food tonight," my father frequently announced when Warner and I were young.)

Photos of the those years show his room decorated with a few souvenirs from Germany. They also show his roommates lounging on their beds in T-shirts and slacks, surrounded by piles of books. There are shots of trips taken with friends in a Volkswagen bus: to Tanglewood (my mother is in one photo, sitting on the roof of the vehicle) and the Cape (only men in the pictures). Obviously, my father occupied his time with more than classes. Intriguingly, under a photo of him with his arm wrapped firmly around the shoulders of a young, slim blond wearing a striped sailor top and tight white pants—she is leaning into him with her head almost resting on his shoulder—he wrote only "Gloucester." In many pictures he is smoking a cigarette or clenching a pipe between his teeth, as in a smiling picture of him in Lexington, clad in a suit and woolen overcoat, a large American flag obscuring most of the background.

At the beginning of his coursework, Hans scraped by painfully, hindered by his lack of formal education in English. On his initial chemistry exam, he spent a great deal of time translating the first question into German and then his own answer back into English. When, feeling triumphant, he moved on to the second question, he was shocked to hear the professor announce that time was up. With amazement and shame, he raised his head and watched the other students hand in their completed examinations before piling out of the room.

But his English improved rapidly. When my mother talked about first meeting him, she always mentioned, in addition to how handsome he looked, that he was the only one in the M.I.T. German student group who did not spend his time talking about Germany. In every way, my father embraced his new country. Fifteen days after getting his Massachusetts driver's license, he purchased a 1949 Chrysler sedan with "37,283 miles on it." Six months later he notes in his diary, "Accident, Main Street, New Haven, Connecticut, 10am." The next year that sedan took him farther, on a trip across the country. The car represented his desire to explore.

In October 1960, my father was granted permanent resident status. It would be almost four years until he defended his doctoral dissertation, and he did not obtain full citizenship until 1970. But as
soon as he arrived in New York, Hans had set his course: new country, new culture, new life.

Perhaps my mother admired this clarity of vision because she
lacked it in herself. When she first arrived in Cambridge, she lived in
a room at the YWCA on Berkeley Street. These cramped and restric-
tive quarters did not suit her, and soon she found a fellow lab technician, a young American woman named Sue, to share a room with
closer to campus. The two seemed to be a good match—both young
women striking out on their own for the first time, both feeling
some trepidation and discontent. Two years later, Sue, then married,
wrote to my mother about her relief at no longer wanting to "go out
in the middle of the street and scream like I used to tell you I did."
My mother, still feeling a strong, insistent pull from her parents, had
her own conflicts during that year. Nevertheless, she extended her
contract with Professor Grant. But in the fall of 1960 surprised all
her new American acquaintances by suddenly moving back to West
Germany.

She did not last long back at home with her dictatorial father and
depressed mother, despite the cheery company of her two youngest
brothers. With her savings from her work in the States, she purchased a new car, a pearl-white VW sedan with a sunroof, and quickly
found employment at another Max Planck Institute, in Stuttgart. Yet
she felt conflicted, even with the relative freedom of having an auto-
mobile and an income. Almost every letter from people she knew in
the States begs to hear something, anything from her. Friends ask
about her future plans, which she describes differently to different
people, from pursuing a PhD, to staying at the institute, to getting
married in Germany. After almost two years of continued oppression
from the domineering atmosphere at home, she became convinced
again that her escape route lay across the ocean. She returned to
Boston with the express goal of finding a husband. Her parents were
pushing her to marry, and by choosing a man who wanted to build

a life in the United States instead of Germany, she could simultaneously fulfill and contradict their wishes. So my mother secured a
job at a private lab in the Boston area and set out on a manhunt.

She had suitors from her previous stay, my father among them.
Accepting several invitations every weekend, she explored many options. Later she confessed that a few of these men probably had more
on their minds than chaste dating, but, my mother explained to me,
her inexperience protected her. Even when she was alone in a man's
room, all the traditional overtures went embarrassingly unnoticed,
until the man disappointedly escorted her home.

Then along came Hans, this time more seriously than before,
and offering her something unique. Seemingly unfettered by his
own heritage, he appeared very American. Self-assured and confident, he broke with tradition. He cooked and drew and worked with
his hands. Rather than suggesting trips to the symphony or dinner
in staid restaurants, he pursued her along unusual lines. "August 2,
1962: Irmgard for dinner at my apartment—I cooked. August 16:
canoe trip with Irmgard in Maine. September 15 and 16: trip with
Irmgard to Vermont," are the entries in my father's diary. And then
on October 25 he wrote her a letter in which he proposed marriage.
Buried deep in the folder of correspondence my mother cataloged as
"Christmas 1961—Engagement 1962" I found his epistle, written in
German:

My dear Irmgard,
This will probably all overtake you so suddenly that you
become scared. But I love you so much that this week
without you seems horrible. Can you forgive me?
    If I could afford it, I would buy airline tickets this
afternoon for Reno, and we would marry tomorrow. Thinking
about this keeps me awake at night. And yet tomorrow I will
only see you in a large group of people.
    I cannot offer you more in this moment than a great
and true love. You probably envisioned something more
dramatic, but life doesn't always go as you think it will. If
we can't marry right away, then I would very much like it if

we were at least engaged as soon as possible. I am afraid to say this to you, because I know you would like more time, and I can be very patient if it is necessary. But is it really necessary?

I love you terribly,

Hans

On October 28 she accepted his proposal.

THE DAY I FOUND these materials in my basement, I sat on the cold linoleum floor, astounded. I examined items until deep into the evening and later spent even more time confronting my misperceptions about my parents. My father's boxes contained meticulously kept files, although I had always known Hans as extremely disorganized. He had written detailed timelines of the important events in every year, giving a bird's-eye view of his experiences from birth until the mid-1980s. My mother, who had always presented herself as having turned her back on the past, saved hundreds of letters to and from her parents, along with at least a hundred more to and from friends and relatives. All these were from the 1950s, '60s, and '70s. I also found her grammar school workbooks and intricate photo collages of her times at the two Max Planck Institutes.

Gradually, I realized, a mystery was unfolding before my eyes. As I closely examined the clues my parents left behind, the identities of two entirely new individuals emerged. Uncovering their histories afforded me a fuller, more three-dimensional understanding of who my parents had been. Complexity and context highlighted the varied facets of their lives, whereas before I had seen only their reflections in the two-dimensional plane of parenthood. In front of me now appeared the dashing, adventurous student, the conflicted, submissive daughter, and most astonishing of all, the exuberant couple in love for the entire world to see.

By complete coincidence, I now lived just outside Boston, where most of my parents' early stories had played out. If I searched, could I find the addresses of their various apartments, scattered around the city? Where had they lived when they were first married? Had they ever been to my current hometown?

The answers had to wait; it was late, and Ron was returning from his conference the next day. But the following Saturday morning, I returned to the basement before breakfast, still wearing pajama bottoms and a T-shirt. As I descended the creaky stairs, I yelled up to Ron before closing the door behind me, "I'm going down here for a few minutes. I just want to take another quick look at my parents' stuff." Four hours later Ron opened the door and called down to inquire about lunch. I still sat on the floor on a fringed brown cushion, mesmerized.

"Come down, Ron. You have to see this!" I exclaimed when he interrupted my reverie. In a minute he was leaning over my shoulder.

"You're never going to believe this," I said. "Look at this. It's my parents' wedding announcement." I handed the photo album over to him from where I sat, holding back the page of thin, spider web–design tissue paper that separated the pages.

"Nice," he said in a voice that conveyed kindness but indifference. "Looks pretty. I'm glad you're having fun down here."

"No," I insisted. I straightened up, bracing one hand on my knee to support my complaining back. Next to him, I balanced the album on my left hand and pointed with my right. "You're not seeing it. Look . . . here. I almost missed it, too, because the whole thing looks like a matted photo."

The front of the announcement displayed a small picture of my mother in her white wedding gown and veil. Just her nose peeked out from behind the mass of white taffeta tumbling from the crown on her head. She was handing her small bouquet of roses to a handsome older man in a tuxedo in front of a car. I had paused at this page when glancing through the album, because this leaf contained only a single photo. Then I had noticed the slight creases in the bottom right-hand corner of the matting. Curious, I had tugged at this area and folded open the card. Inside, printed on one side in German and the other in English, was my parents' wedding announcement.

"Nice," Ron said again, when I showed him.

"No," I contradicted again. "Don't you see now? The address?"

"It's some church in Waltham."

"The *other* address. Where they lived. Look—89 Northbury Road. In Concord! My parents moved to Concord right after they got married. Can you believe it? Right near where we live now. Isn't that amazing?"

Ron caught some of my excitement. "Let's go upstairs and Google the address. I think that's a street right in the center of town."

Their street branched off Concord's main thoroughfare near the library. We had, in fact, been down the same road a number of times before—we'd even walked along it.

"Let's go there on our bikes this afternoon," Ron suggested. "We'll take our camera, and I can take a picture of you standing in front of your parents' old home."

My anticipation increased as later that day we bicycled along the narrow path leading through woods and marshes to Concord. I thought along the way of the album. To my knowledge, my mother had taken all the older family albums in the divorce. Yet although the organization and pasting of the photos showed my mother's careful hand, I had found the album in my father's belongings. Had she deliberately left it behind when she moved out, not wanting to be reminded of the joyful times? Or had my father insisted on keeping it?

The arrangement of the pictures told a story. After pages and pages of crowded wedding and reception shots, the tone suddenly shifted to one of lovers' intimacy. My father shaving around his post-wedding goatee in the bathroom, his wavy hair tousled, a towel around his neck. My father sitting at a picnic table under a tree in the backyard, having pancakes, orange juice, and coffee served in elegant white china, the seats opposite him occupied by two Siamese cats. My mother in sweatpants and a hooded sweatshirt, obviously braless, watering the garden. Both of them in lawn chairs, reading. The back of my mother's head as she canoes on the Concord River. Car trouble at a house on Cape Cod. And my favorite: my mother, again in the sweatshirt, sitting in a passenger seat outside a lodge, holding a map and smiling at the photographer with delight.

In my lifetime, I never saw such love, contentment, trust, and repose intermingled in her features.

As we approached Northbury Road, my excitement mounted. The house in the photos had been white clapboard, with a white picket fence and a small garden in the back. *Will I recognize it?* We turned off the main street. Ron began calling out numbers as we passed houses. "Eighteen . . . Twenty-nine." Large, regal residences commanded either side of the road. Well maintained and tastefully painted with contrasting trim, they exuded New England charm while also emanating old-money confidence. Porches enveloped their fronts and sides, upper-floor windows were dormered, lawns were manicured. I remembered my mother telling me that she and my father had once house-sat for a professor on sabbatical. Nothing else could explain how a newly married graduate student and lab technician could afford to live out here.

"Sixty-three . . . Seventy-five," Ron called out. I held my breath. And then, "Ninety-nine?" We both braked.

"How's that possible?" I asked.

I checked over my left shoulder for traffic and made a U-turn. Riding back toward town more slowly, I looked again. Yes, that was ninety-nine. And yes, farther up, that was seventy-five. Which could only mean . . .

As I turned my bicycle around again, I saw Ron already standing in front of it, laughing.

"No way!" I protested.

Chapter 5

Talking in the Kitchen

2008, 1993, 1983

Ron, who has a dry wit, exulted. "Yes, Sweetie, here it is. The only dump in all of Concord: your parents' former home!"

We stood staring at the front of the house. No wonder we had missed it on our first pass. You had to look closely to make out the façade through the tangle of trees, brush, and vines grown up around it. Someone had boarded up the lower windows. The roof looked as though it might cave in. "Condemned" signs should have been plastered over all the entrances.

I was in shock. On the ride over I had imagined myself walking up to the front door of the white house and knocking. I pictured the owners graciously welcoming me in and taking me on a tour of my ancestral home. I would see the bathroom where my father had posed, the kitchen where he and my mother had cooked, the bedroom where they had slept. I would breathe the air and admire the view. At last I would be visiting the site of my own beginnings.

Startling me out of my reverie, Ron ran around me with a camera. "Pose as though you're going in. Point to the entrance," he exhorted, eager to capture the situation in all its absurdity. I glared at him in annoyance.

Then I felt my stomach begin to shake as a comic epiphany burst out of me. "This is *perfect*!" I laughed. "It's exactly the way it should be."

I had been looking for a closing of the loop and now had found it. Exactly what happened between my parents after they left Concord will forever remain a mystery. But as a child, I had not experienced the joy I had seen in those photos. Instead, I had witnessed the emotional disintegration of their marriage. The crumbling house where my parents lived for only a year before I was conceived became a powerful metaphor for all the things I had intuited about their relationship but had never been able to articulate.

IN 1993, AT AGE twenty-seven, I returned from where I was living at the time to my father's home in Wilmington. As usual during a visit, my father and I spent many hours together in the kitchen. That bright yellow room where the wallpaper admonished, "You are what you eat!" was in every sense the heart of his house, the place where friends met, parties began, and most conversations started.

Hans showed love through the preparation of food, as his mother had done before him. No one he cared about could enter his house without being asked, "Would you like something to eat?" And if you knew him well, you understood this wasn't really a question. "No, thank you" would be countered with "How about something to drink?" or "Just a little snack?" or "Why don't we go sit down—I'll make us some tea while we talk." You would be eating or drinking something before long.

Soon after our family moved to the house in Wilmington, Hans remodeled the kitchen. He chose at that time, the mid-seventies, a canary color theme. But he selected the unusual wallpaper for its price as much as for its shade. It had slight printing defects, and Hans found it among the other rolls of "bargains." I spent many mornings preparing my school lunch while sleepily staring at the slightly overlapping lettering: "Youre what yoeat!"

I grew up in this house with two men. After my mother moved into an apartment down the street (this was literally true—even with our small strides, Warner and I could walk there in ten minutes), our family essentially became a threesome. My mother called us children every day, and we spent three weekends out of four with her, but day-to-day living for Warner and me revolved around my father. On top of his full-time job, Hans cooked our meals, washed our clothes, took us to the doctor, painted our bedrooms, and even sewed our curtains.

Hans often remarked that he did not know why Irmgard had left.

Irmgard maintained that she moved out because her relationship with Hans had irreversibly deteriorated. She could no longer live with him and be a good mother to us, she insisted. Unfortunately for me, she chose as her main example of maternal failure the story of my dropping a dinner plate on the kitchen floor. "I yelled at Tina for doing that and afterwards couldn't believe it. I never yelled at the children about accidents. That was exactly the moment I knew that I had to move out." My nine-year-old mind grasped that story's unmistakable and deeply disturbing logic: *My breaking a plate made Mom leave.* Unintentionally, my mother's tale, coupled with the actual fallout of the divorce, established a chain of causal connections that became well traveled in my brain: *My mother can always leave me again, and if she does, it will be my fault.*

Outsiders, even friends and relatives—even my *mother's* relatives—bemoaned the situation at the time. "How can a mother abandon her young children?" they muttered under their breath. "Poor Hans. What a saint he is to take care of those two. She should be ashamed of herself." It did not help Warner and me to hear these accusations. We were naturally loyal to both our parents. And, truthfully, *neither* of them was a saint. Each carried a share of the responsibility for the failed marriage and for the repercussions.

In the years after the divorce, Warner and I were left on our own to a greater extent than modern psychology might recommend. And abandonment played a role in the relationships he and I developed with Irmgard and Hans from that point on. We did not have either of them available to us in the ways we needed. Irmgard called and wrote us notes and tried to make the weekends with us as much fun as possible, but children live in the present. And she was not present.

On the other side, the burden of caretaking overwhelmed Hans, and he shut down at the first sign of an emotional escalation between my brother and me. He would boom at us in his huge voice to stop fighting and then retreat to his bedroom, slamming a door somewhere along the way.

As many other children do, Warner and I learned to live on our own, in a world of fighting and truces, games and tears. Like a number of our childhood acquaintances, after the divorce we walked ourselves to school in the mornings and came home to an empty house in the afternoons. My father's attempt at hiring an afternoon babysitter for his eight- and nine-year-old kids failed miserably. We decided instantly we didn't need anyone to watch us, especially not the person my father had found, a slightly awkward teenage boy too gullible for his own good.

The pitiable fellow became the target of all our pent-up anger and frustration. After complaining vociferously to Hans about not needing a sitter, Warner and I took matters into our own hands, colluding to prove to him that we would be fine alone in the house. One rainy afternoon we ran into the kitchen shouting about a large dog we'd seen in our driveway. "We're scared! Can you go out and make it go away?" we pleaded movingly. No sooner had the boy run outside to shoo the animal away than—click—we locked the back door behind him. He pounded on it for a while, asking to be let in, but then he gave up and went home. *No way is this worth two fifty an hour,* he must have thought.

Hans decided not to find a replacement. So Warner and I had the hours between three and five as a private, unsupervised pause in our lives. We often played together inside, constructing elaborate forts from the black-and-white-checked living room couch cushions and wooden end tables, draping spare bedsheets over our constructions to make the interior more private. Or we read beloved books in our separate rooms. But our brawls stand out most to me from that period: chasing each other around the house; Hans coming home to broken artwork and yelling; my running like a demon after Warner through the backyard, ready to pull his hair out. Luckily, we never sustained anything more than bruises from a well-landed punch or two. Despite my omnipresent fury, I also hesitated to inflict damage on Warner, and he had the same reluctance. Because in addition to being each other's foremost rivals, we were also each other's foremost playmates. We competed at Monopoly for hours on end, played kickball with the neighborhood children, and read together in our secret hideout in the attic. We raced around the streets on our bicycles and engaged in badminton tournaments in the yard. But we never eluded the rage, anger, and resentment for long.

Over the passing years, we each made our own peace with the divorce and developed our own styles of interacting with each other. Hans and Irmgard also constructed a superficial and fragile armistice. Weekends with my mother eventually condensed into long Friday night dinners at the same restaurant, where we always sat at the same table, ordered the same food, and talked for hours. The continuity comforted us. Sometimes afterward Warner and I spent the night at her place.

Hans continued taking frequent business trips of several days or more, leaving us in the care of a sitter when he was away longer. By the time we were in our mid-teens, he left us alone at home. Hans returned home to fewer and fewer casualties of sibling rivalry. With a lessening of his financial worries and our growing independence and willingness to share in the responsibilities of the house, Hans relaxed. We harvested vegetables together at a victory garden on the outskirts of town during long summer evenings, where, more often than we helped pick tomatoes, Warner and I ran off after butterflies to add to our small and repetitive collection. But this didn't bother the calmer Hans.

Because of random school district lines and desegregation, Warner and I attended different schools for several years. In high school our paths merged again. In the intervening period, Warner had skipped a year, and we found ourselves sharing most of the same classes.

In separate schools, we had enjoyed eight hours of respite from each other every day. In high school, we were forced to be together for almost all our waking hours. Try as we might, we could not avoid each other's company.

Our school was no exception in having the usual breakdown of students into overlapping subgroups. Warner and I both gravitated to the nerds. We started to see each other in situations we had never before contemplated. *Warner has some good-looking friends*, I realized. *Tina hangs out with girls I'd like to date*, Warner thought. As our social circles blended, we did as well, and our once tempestuous relationship began to mature. By senior year I proudly called my brother my best friend.

Familiarity, in our case, bred not contempt but understanding and respect. Now in close proximity for our entire days, we could no longer exaggerate our triumphs. And we could no longer hide from each other the typical wounds teenage psyches sustain. I remember the turning point—when I felt victimized by a number of former friends. Because I had committed some unpardonable sin, such as sitting with the wrong people in the cafeteria, they had ousted me from their group and made hurtful comments about me behind my back. Instead of standing up to them, I meekly swallowed their abuse, and for a few weeks Warner watched me skip lunch and take circuitous routes through the high school corridors.

Then one evening he said, "Tina, let's take a walk."

In the early dusk of fall, we strolled the few blocks from home to a small playground we had frequented a decade earlier. Walking, we discussed classes, movies, and plans for college. Then we sat on the swings, swaying gently in the twilight and not saying much. After a few minutes, Warner braked, took off the backpack he had been wearing, reached inside, and handed me a folded jacket.

"What's this?" I asked.

"I got it for you. It's a jeans jacket."

Speechless, I shook it out and tried it on. It fit perfectly.

"You look good," Warner said, as he pushed himself close to me so that he could flip up the collar. "You look tough."

"I can't believe it," I responded, sitting up taller. "I don't have anything like this." The stiff material strained slightly against any movement. It felt like a protective armor. I thought of the kids in school who wore jackets like this, kids for whom everyone had grudging respect.

I slid off the swing and strutted around, hands in the jacket pockets, head held a bit higher than usual.

"Yeah," smiled Warner. "I thought you could use a little help. Nobody's going to mess with you if you've got that on."

Once my nemesis, my brother had begun looking out for me.

During that senior year, when Hans left town, Warner and I sat in the yellow kitchen over plates of noodles for dinner, making each other laugh until we had to spit the food out for fear of choking. We wrote our college essays together at the same table, occasionally reading sentences aloud. We studied there for our finals. And after graduation we got drunk there with a genial, sandy-haired classmate, taking Hans up on his progressive yet fatherly suggestion that, if we had to drink alcohol, we should do it in the safety of our house.

My father hardly imbibed at all, but he had accumulated an assortment of liquor for the parties he loved to host. On the occasion of our graduation, we lined up all the bottles on the kitchen table in order of height—rum, vodka, gin, amaretto, Cointreau—and poured ourselves a small glass of each. With that mixture churning around inside us, we only narrowly escaped getting seriously sick to our stomachs. We did have a hard time getting up the stairs. When we finally went to bed, Warner confiscated our friend's car keys, to make sure he didn't get any inebriated ideas.

Sunshine streamed through my window late the following morning, rousing me from my heavy slumber. Only Speedy's hungry meowing downstairs broke the silence. I got up to knock on Warner's door. As I passed the guest room, I saw that our friend had already left.

"When did he go?" I asked Warner, who was still under the covers.

"I made him do a calculus problem at four a.m., to make sure he was fit to drive. Then I gave him back his car keys," Warner mumbled and pulled the sheets over his head.

I smiled at the thought of the two of them being able to do math at that hour—our friend doing the problem and Warner knowing the correct answer. If my leaving had depended on that ability *any* day, I would have had been under permanent house arrest.

"Thanks for looking out for him," I said, but Warner had already turned over and gone back to sleep.

OVER A DECADE LATER, in 1993, during my brief visit home, Hans made smoked salmon sandwiches for our lunch. He welcomed me back with food, as always. As he sliced through the shiny orange fish, I thought about everything that had transpired in that room. I thought about where we all had been, and where each of us was going. I looked again at the overlapping lettering on the wallpaper, which had been a persistent reminder that we are affected in no small measure by the choices we make in life.

By that time I already knew about the choices my mother intended to make and how she planned to face old age. *But what about Hans?*

Throughout my childhood, I had been indoctrinated by my mother to "expect the worst" in any situation. Although by nature an optimist, from her I had learned fatalism to guard against dashed expectations. When you expect the worst, you're less likely to be disappointed. But this outlook does make for a jumpy existence. If someone I love doesn't come home from a party on time, the possibility of a car accident looms large in my mind. If the phone rings at three a.m., my heart's pounding has less to do with the shock of being awoken than with the multiple scenarios of family disaster that electrify my sleepy eyes.

Hans abhorred this catastrophe-based thinking. "Why contemplate the possibility of rain when the sun is shining now?" he maintained. Fundamentally, Hans loved living. Like everyone else, he made plans and looked forward to or worried about the future, but the commotion of daily life most occupied his mind. He devoted huge amounts of energy to activities he truly enjoyed, eagerly distributing the tangible products of his labors to his children or his friends. He expected that his plans would work out well, and he carried things through based on this hopeful principle. He usually did not allow small setbacks to frustrate him for long.

But in many ways I took after my mother. I expected the worst, including about Hans's future. While I sat hungrily at the kitchen table that afternoon, I extrapolated the wallpaper's admonition to retirement planning: "You are in later years what you plan for now." As morbid as I found her arrangements, I could not fault my mother in the preparation department. She had her retirement plans neatly laid out: permanent retirement.

Hans, although older than my mother, lagged behind. From my relatively youthful perspective, he seemed to be well over the hill of life. I was beginning to panic on his behalf. Plans should be made for the inevitable as well as the unknown, I thought. *What if something happens to him without his having made provisions?* He always declared he would make arrangements to take care of himself. I knew he intended to move into the Quaker retirement community, where continuing care would be available no matter what his needs. *But when?*

Of course, Hans was preparing for retirement at a pace completely consistent with *his* outlook on life, not mine. And compared to many people, he was making sensible plans. He wanted to move of his own volition into a community of older people. He looked forward to reveling in the freedom from household chores that living in an apartment would provide. He knew that a "continuing care community" would liberate him from the repairs that living in a house built in 1923 required. The retirement community Hans had chosen required prospective residents to pass a test of their cognitive and physical independence. So he would not postpone the decision forever. He would move while he was still fit, enabling himself to have as much autonomy as possible while he still had the stamina to live life on his own. If he ever needed assisted living or nursing home care, the community offered those services as well.

Of course, one has many alternatives to moving into such a place if help is needed for survival. Staying at home and having aides come in, relying on relatives and friends, or moving directly into assisted living or nursing home facilities only begin to describe the choices. But Hans preferred the least risky option. Well in advance of any emergency, he put his name on the "inactive" list of the Quaker Community. This placed him in a holding position until the time when he decided to become "active" and search for an apartment unit. He felt comfortable with this arrangement.

Nevertheless, I could not see the future from my father's standpoint. What seemed utterly sensible to him seemed foolhardy to me. I was too young to realize how different the world felt from his perspective at sixty-two—how short his life may have seemed to him and how much he yet wanted to do. As far as I was concerned, my father was playing Russian roulette with his future. Home on this visit for only a couple of days, I wanted to push him to make some decisions while I was around.

Hans concentrated on the task at hand, preparing the salmon sandwiches. I pressed ahead with my sudden agenda.

"So, Hans, you know that I'm planning on moving back to this area for graduate school in a few years," I began the conversation, as my father stood at the counter.

"Yes, Tina," he said, turning to smile at me while holding the fish knife. "But I wish you were going to stay here longer than just two years. You've been gone so long already."

"I know you do." The conversation had managed to turn immediately toward a point of constant strain between us. Hans took my decision to move back to the area only temporarily as a slight. I knew this, and tried to steer for neutral ground.

"I'll be here for a while anyway, and who knows what will happen in the meantime?"

Hans washed his hands in the sink and placed the sandwiches on the table. He sat down. I began again, this time approaching the issue of retirement head-on.

"You're still on the list at the Quaker Community, aren't you?"

"Yes, as far as I know." Nothing in his tone of voice indicated surprise at the abrupt change of topic. "I gave them a lot of money for that privilege. They'd better hold up their end of the deal," he joked while chewing.

"Have you talked to them about it lately, about how long it would take to move to the 'active' list?" I believed this was the key step in making a decision. Otherwise Hans could remain inactive for years on end.

Hans glanced up at me between mouthfuls. "No, I haven't even thought about it. I just put my name on the list a few years ago. The time to start thinking about the last part of my life is still so far away. You know I am just starting up my new business. I'd be crazy to move out of this house for another ten or fifteen years, at least. I am too busy to think about retiring out in the countryside!"

"But you'll keep your name on the list, right?"

"I don't think it gets removed unless you ask them. But I'm not completely sure what I want to do yet. I like this house." He paused, looking around the kitchen wistfully. "Maybe I should look into staying here when the time comes."

I could feel his discomfort with the conversation, but that did not deter me. Suddenly I had a vision of him lying on the kitchen floor, permanently incapacitated by a heart attack.

As though he read my thoughts, Hans laughed and asked, "Are you worried that I might keel over tomorrow?"

"No." I paused. "But you never know . . ."

Hans's voice became serious, and the sparkle faded from his eyes. "Tina, I'm not ready to make any decisions about this kind of thing yet. You know I have been going to a lot of trainings to get my business up and running. I'm starting it from scratch. I've invested a lot of time and money into it. I'm not ready to retire. I'm just beginning. And I'm not ready to move."

He paused to take a long look at me and then continued. "I *am* planning on staying healthy. This is my decision, you know. I'll make it when I am ready, and I don't think I'm being irresponsible. I'm in good shape."

He was not angry with me, but I understood the message. He had finished talking about this topic. And so, outwardly, I agreed with him, nodding my head and concentrating again on my sandwich.

To myself, I expressed my concerns. *You're making a potential mistake, Hans. You don't live with anyone who can take care of you. No one will call an ambulance if you fall in the bathtub and can't get to a phone. You had that small heart attack eight years ago. You could have another one at any time. Sixty-two is too early to move out of here, I agree. But waiting until you're well into your seventies could be too late.*

Yet I had to admit to myself that he had the right to make his own decision. Even in retrospect, I credit myself with no ability to prophesy. My panic at that time about Hans's possible decline had mainly to do with my own internal struggles about death and dying, primarily influenced by my mother's plans. I feared for Hans mostly because I feared for myself. I envied Hans the luxury of simply enjoying the present without worrying too much about the future. Death was approaching me, in the person of my mother. Although the event was still far off, it riveted me and at the same time left me feeling incredibly unprepared.

Chapter 6

Making Plans

2003

When my mother and I talked about her plans, the conversations frequently repeated themselves. I knew she was serious, and I thought long and hard about the most logical arguments I could make to try and dissuade her. But she had a response for everything.

Me: "Killing yourself would be unfair to Warner and me."

Irmgard: "You only think that now. When the time comes, you'll be relieved you don't need to care for an incontinent, senile old woman."

Me: "You are healthy and would live healthily much past seventy."

Irmgard: "That may be true, but I don't want to take any chances. It's always better to leave a party early, when no one wants you to go, than to stay until you're kicked out."

Me: "I cannot, or at the very least do not want to, live without you, and ending your life prematurely will deprive us of wonderful experiences we can have together."

Irmgard: "We can work on having wonderful experiences now. It has to end sometime."

Me: "Killing yourself is selfish."

Irmgard: "Yes, I'm doing this for myself. But I'm also doing it for both of you. You are too young to understand, but someday you'll be glad I did it this way."

Me: "You can wait until you are really sick and do it then."

Irmgard: "If I thought I would have all my wits about me no matter what happens to my body, I'd do that. But you never know how it's going to happen. I could have a stroke and then have dementia, or become a vegetable, or lose the ability to move my arms, and then it would be too late to take matters into my own hands. I'm not a risk taker."

Me: "I love you. Please don't do it."

Irmgard: "I love you and have the highest respect for you, Tina. But I'm going to do it anyway."

Invariably, she held her ground. And when we talked, at the end of our discussion I usually circled back toward the same question: "When?"

"Do you *really* want to know?" my mother would ask slowly. She would look at me with compassion. I could sense that some small part of her knew that, while this decision gave her a sense of ultimate peace, it inflicted upon me terrible pain.

"No," I said softly. She was correct. "I don't want to know exactly when. It's before seventy, but not any time soon, right? It's not for years, right?"

"No, Tina, not for years."

My mother's plan originated with her sense of the precariousness of health and life. Believing she had some measure of control calmed her. But she was dragging me, an unwilling participant, into a process about which she did not want to engage in meaningful dialogue. For her own reasons, she wanted me to know of her plans but to stand as a detached observer, regarding her preparations as if looking through a window, untouched and uninvolved.

This would prove impossible.

PEOPLE WHO KNEW MY mother well described her as eccentric. People who knew my father well often described him as a Renaissance man. My independent, extremely focused mother enjoyed the small, quiet things in life. My dashing, multitalented father never lacked for grand and interesting things to do.

From my early childhood, home improvement projects occupied Hans's evenings and weekends. None of them had much to do with his job as an engineer. Perhaps he enjoyed them more because of that. When Warner and I attended summer camp, we received letters detailing the progress of the upstairs bathroom or bedroom remodeling. To show us we were missed, he signed these letters for Speedy and our pet gerbils, pressing the animals' paws onto an ink pad and then onto the page. Sometimes a gerbil got away and peppered the letter with tiny black scratches signaling a futile dash toward freedom.

We returned home to find black and white tile, new carpeting, or refinished woodwork. He took on the small backyard, progressively shrinking the middle patch of grass by planting irises and peonies near the house as well as tomatoes, zucchini, cucumbers, and peppers along the fence. Over the years, as the summer vegetable and flower gardens expanded, the area of grass left in the center became so small that it no longer allowed for kickball or badminton. Only Speedy was still thrilled by the narrow strip of green.

My mother excelled at doing one thing at a time, slowly but astonishingly well, including the upkeep of her living quarters. She never broke any dishes, because she never had conversations while cleaning out the dishwasher and never rushed through clearing the table. Her appliances rarely failed, because she always read the instruction books, using a bright pink highlighter to underline the recommendations regarding routine maintenance. She flushed the insides of the iron with distilled water every six months to clean out any deposits. She ran the air conditioning periodically in winter to keep the mechanism lubricated, bundling herself in a winter coat and ski pants to keep warm.

Hans, on the other hand, was the consummate multitasker. When he answered the phone, he headed straight into the living room or kitchen to start doing something else. Talking did not occupy enough of his mind, so he watered the plants or rummaged around in the refrigerator for dinner ingredients. To facilitate his mobility, he equipped all the telephones in our house with extra-long cords. When cordless technology greatly extended his roaming ability, I found us having conversations with the strangest background noises. I didn't dare ask where he was. Bathroom, roof, or street—only signal strength limited his range.

Always eager to avoid distractions, my mother taught me the

value of giving someone your undivided attention. During a telephone conversation, she sat down in a chair and faced away from the window. She switched the radio, TV, or CD player off. And, unlike Hans, she would remember exactly what you said.

Although they both grew up during the war, my mother spent her money carefully on a small number of high-quality items she used for decades, while Hans concerned himself primarily with price. If pressed for a reason, when his frugality pushed the limits of what most people would classify as sensible, he explained that his family had suffered horrible deprivations during his childhood. Irmgard believed "you get what you pay for" and wanted the best, even if this meant doing without until she had saved enough to afford it. Hans did not easily part with his money and went out of his way for any bargain. He also enjoyed the challenge of building something from scratch and whenever possible would do that rather than purchase the object in a store.

For holidays Hans made a festive German drink, *Feuerzangenbowle*. A large, hard cone made entirely of sugar was an essential ingredient, but it cost five dollars at the neighborhood German delicatessen. So in the evenings he returned to his lab, where he ran experiments during the day. In the era before corporate cost cutting, others also certainly took advantage of their employers, but I imagine Hans was the only one using company resources to compress grains of sugar.

Creating the mold, according to the story he would often tell, did not present the main challenge, although it had to be constructed so that he could easily remove the finished product. The problem was getting the sugar to stick together in any shape at all. This had to be done under considerable pressure, because for a successful drink, the sugar had to hold together long enough to absorb some alcohol and be set on fire. My father, despite enlisting the help of coworkers in the machine shop and elsewhere, just couldn't design a machine to apply enough force.

Five dollars to buy the thing in the store down the street, or hundreds of dollars and countless hours spent to try and make it yourself? Typically motivated by parsimony, Hans simply enjoyed the process of *trying* to save money. Only after failing countless times in the lab did he purchase with great reluctance the precious cones. He grumbled each time he brought one out of hiding at a holiday. "How do they make this hold together so well? It can't be that difficult." He would hold it up close to his eyes for inspection, as though if he just stared long and hard enough, he would be able to decipher the mysterious bonding technique. Then he enjoyed the costly privilege of setting it alight.

TEN YEARS AFTER THE first conversation we had about retirement, Hans and I again sat at his kitchen table. It was 2003, and to both my parents' delight, my move back to Wilmington had become permanent. I treasured being in such close proximity to them both again. Living only blocks from each of them, I took advantage of every opportunity to develop our relationships. I also wanted to spend as much time with my mother as possible. She was then in her late sixties, and her countdown was reverberating loudly in my mind.

As usual, Hans and I conversed over food.

"What did you put in this lentil soup? It's amazing!" I enthused, eagerly spooning more of the rich broth into my mouth.

"Well," he mused, "lentils?"

"No, seriously, can you write down the recipe for me? I want to make this at home."

"You know me. It's always just a mix of what I have in the fridge. Today I had some extra carrots. Oh, and there was also a box of leftover Chinese take-out that was going to go bad if I didn't use it. So I threw it in too."

"Well, I wouldn't have thought of it, but brilliant idea."

"I'm glad you like it. You know how I cook. It's just serendipity." He waved his hand in the air.

"I'll take the leftovers home if you'll let me. I could eat this forever."

Hans nodded in agreement. "It sure beats the food at the Quaker Community. I don't know how my friends stand it out there. I went to visit some of them the other day and the lunch was terrible. At least there's a salad bar now, but the vegetables were so overcooked."

Hans had strict ideas about food that stemmed from his mother, the wartime scarcities they had endured, and his personal proclivities. Food should be delicious, inexpensive, and interesting. It should also be prepared in his own kitchen.

"Well, Hans, few places can meet *your* standards," I said. "But when you move out there, you won't have to eat every meal in the common dining room. You'll still have a kitchen."

Then I jumped at the chance to interject some questions about his plans for retirement. "By the way, have you thought any more about moving onto their active list lately?"

"No, Tina, I'm not ready to move yet." Frugality reared its familiar head as he continued. "The basic units are so small, and the larger ones are so expensive. I'm not made of money, you know. Even if I sell the house, they still require a huge down payment, and then they want a fat check every month on top of that."

"Well, it might not be as bad as it seems. Do you know the exact figures?"

"Yes. I have the brochure upstairs in my files."

"When did you get that?" I asked, taken aback. The last time we had discussed this subject, Hans was not aware of any details and seemed reluctant to investigate.

"They sent me a postcard about an informational event a month or so ago. I went. It was really interesting. But I told them I was just checking things out."

I could imagine Hans having been quite forceful about not wanting to be pressured into committing prematurely. But his having spontaneously taken another step closer to moving elated me. "That's great!" I enthused but then found myself at a loss for words. *How do I help him in this process, when he's just clearly stated that he doesn't want to be pushed? What leverage do I have to make him see that sooner might be better than later?*

Flustered, I blurted out the first thing that came to my mind,

"You're seventy-two, after all. I'm sure you're reaching the average age when people start moving in there."

In hindsight, probably not the way to broach the subject.

"Why do you always say that I'm getting old? I think the average age of people there is something like eighty, and they said that people there actually live ten years longer." He spoke rapidly, citing the same arguments I had heard year after year. When he had rattled off the list, he concluded, "So I'm in no rush. I don't want to sell this house yet, and I don't want to quit my business. I'm not ready to become an old person living out in the boondocks. I like living here in the city."

"I know," I responded in a conciliatory voice. I understood his position; part of me even agreed. But I couldn't let go of the central issue, the one that nagged at me constantly: "But you never know what's going to happen. And you do live alone. And you have had a heart attack . . ."

Hans rose and strode to the bookshelf between the kitchen and dining room. He returned with a volume on "reversing heart disease" and placed it on the table between us. He wasn't angry, but he clearly did not accept my point of view.

"Tina," he said, "that was eighteen years ago. You know I have been living carefully, and I believe what this author writes. I watch what I eat and I exercise. You seem determined to kick me into an early grave, but I believe I am healthy. I'm probably in better shape now than when I had the damn heart attack."

"Hans." My eyes filled with tears. "Don't misunderstand me. I am just worried about you, and I don't want you to end up in a bad situation."

Genuinely surprised, he asked, "Tina, if *I'm* not worried, why are you?" He walked over toward me and stretched out his arms. I rose and hugged him.

"This is my decision to make, and I don't think I'm being unreasonable. I am just not ready to do this yet. I have too much else going on."

Against his shoulder I nodded my head. My father also had a clear idea of what was right for him. I knew he would enjoy his life in the retirement community once he acclimated and began participating in the vibrant social life there. But the choice of when to go would be his.

Five years later, searching through Hans's belongings in my basement, I discovered his "Personal Information Form" from the intake materials of the Quaker Community. Among other entries, he had written answers to various questions. The proudest moment of his life? Children graduating from high school and college. The saddest moment of his life? Good friends dying. Frustrations? The need to slow down on activities, and spending so much time sorting and disposing of his things. Why he considered moving to the community? Not wanting to be a burden to his children. And how his children viewed his moving to the community? His daughter urging him to get on with it.

All along, I thought I had been talking to someone with a deaf ear. In reality, *I* was the one who had not listened.

Just as my mother did not want to listen to me.

Chapter 7

Repairing the Past

1996, 2003

Even when I was a child, part of me approved of my parents' decision to divorce. Countless nights I awoke, startled by Irmgard and Hans screaming at each other. I cowered under the covers, hearing only snatches of German.

"Du hast das schon immer getan!" ("You've always done that kind of thing!")

"Why won't you calm down?"

"Why won't you listen?"

"I can't go on like this . . ."

Finally I would crawl halfway down the stairs in tears, peer through the banister, and beg them to stop. Even as an eight-year-old I had a sense of how pathetic I looked sobbing uncontrollably, "Please, Mommy and Daddy . . . Stop fighting! . . . Please!"

It mystified me that my obvious suffering did not persuade them to stop.

Watching them heedlessly tear into each other and rip our family apart from the inside made their eventual separation welcome.

By the time I returned to Wilmington to attend graduate school in 1996, my mother and I had not lived in the same house for twenty-three years. So we embraced the opportunity to get to know each other as adults and took the unorthodox step of choosing to live together again. We hoped it would give us an opportunity to experience some of what we'd missed after she had moved out when I was nine.

My mother and I took on the challenge of sharing the same space for, as we told everyone, "just a year." My father and brother bet against us, convinced we were too similar and too set in our own ways to make a success of such a risky experiment.

In secret, I had another reason for moving in with her and for being determined to make things work between us. I understood her suicide plans only in the vaguest terms. I did not know her exact date, not even the year. But the knowledge that at some point she did not intend to be around never left my mind. I wanted to be close to her. I wanted to get to know her better while I still could. And I wanted to have the chance to talk her out of it, or at least into postponing it.

Much had changed about my mother since she left her marriage. When she moved in with my father, she was young, conflicted, and unsure of herself. She had escaped her family but had not yet found herself. After they were married, my father dictated forceful letters to Irmgard's father, outlining the new boundaries of Irmgard's life. The epistles demanded that she be shown a copy of her father's will, that she be included in family decision making, that the grandchildren be welcomed. Irmgard dutifully typed up the testimonials and signed them, keeping yellow carbon copies of some of the early correspondence. How her father must have fumed at the changes marriage had wrought in his daughter!

In the first years, Irmgard looked to Hans as a role model for independence and self-confidence. She observed him carefully and must have felt protected by the shadow of his strong personality. Hans brimmed with self-reliance and self-assurance. Then Warner and I were born, and business trip after business trip took Hans more and more often away from home. Raising toddlers occupied all Irmgard's time, but it did not consume her mind. Following the path Hans had started to lead her down, she contemplated what *she* wanted out of life. And she realized that she also had goals to achieve.

They had moved to Toledo, Ohio, after my father got his PhD. He worked at Owens Illinois, engineering tiny ceramic tiles used for small transistors in radios and televisions. Irmgard joined neighborhood groups, made friends, and gained confidence. When the women's liberation movement began to trickle even into midwestern suburbia in the late 1960s, my mother soaked up its ideology like a dry sponge. Its values of self-worth and autonomy mirrored her own. Oblivious to the changes taking place in his wife, my father continued to travel and to work on solo projects in the basement. Meanwhile, in between taking us to the zoo and cleaning the house, Irmgard reassessed her situation. She decided she wanted something more.

Irmgard would later describe her initial experiments with self-determination as haphazard. She began to see the fetters her family had placed on her during her youth as if for the first time. Exulting in testing her own limits, she took a few classes, aiming for a college degree, since her German training had no official equivalent in the States. She first enrolled at a nearby community college. Later, when Warner and I began school and she had more time to herself, she attended a university farther away. At encounter groups and in transcendental meditation classes, my mother developed friendships with people who encouraged her to leave Hans. In particular, she met one woman who felt trapped in her marriage. They became close, and this fellow frustrated homemaker fueled my mother's anti-Hans sentiments, although photos in our albums also document her innocently smiling at Hans during dinner parties and laughing with him as he pushes us children on the garden swing set.

Finally, and perhaps most damaging to the marriage, my mother had a number of short-lived extramarital affairs. Irmgard was vague about the exact number, and I never wanted to hear the lurid details. But from what I gathered, she had brief flings with scientists she had known in Germany, or with men she met at the encounter groups. I'm not certain whether Hans knew or suspected, but from what Irmgard said to me over the years, I don't think he did. I will never know for sure, but Hans seems to have been oblivious to many potential signs that the marriage was not moving in a good direction. Responsibilities at the office certainly burdened him. And at home numerous solitary hobbies consumed him, including woodworking, which he excelled at. During those years, he constructed a large jungle gym and sandbox for our backyard, a sewing cabinet with a built-in, flip-up sewing machine for my mother's workroom, a harpsichord for our living room, and a small sailboat for our vacations. Apparently, this left little time for Irmgard and no opportunity to notice she was pulling away.

The person I knew as my mother was born during that time. The submissive daughter transformed herself into an opinionated and determined woman. When Owens Illinois closed its ceramics division in Ohio, Hans found a new position with DuPont in Wilmington. By that point, my mother had secretly determined to divorce.

At Irmgard's insistence, Hans arranged for DuPont to hire her as well. She wanted her own income before she made her final move toward independence. When Hans asked her to do the advance house hunting, she willingly flew to Wilmington without him. She selected a house within a mile of DuPont and our schools but also within walking distance of a number of apartment complexes. She knew she'd be moving out soon and wanted to be sure she would have a place nearby.

A year after we relocated, she announced to Hans her decision to leave. From her description of Hans's reaction, I'd have to say it came as a complete surprise to him.

It certainly surprised Warner and me.

AFTER THE DIVORCE, I never completely trusted Irmgard not to abandon me again. Her determination to end her life prematurely only exacerbated this underlying insecurity. Yet my mother and I maintained a strong bond throughout my childhood, adolescence, and young adulthood. Although not a daily presence in my life, Irmgard made a consistent effort to have as much contact as I would allow. And I appreciated her respect for me and found comfort in her affection.

We understood each other—two independent females. In actuality, she had *chosen* her independence; I had mine forced on me. But the mutual self-reliance of thought and action drew us continually closer as we each matured. When I moved back to Wilmington as an adult, living together to get to know each other better seemed like an entirely reasonable proposal.

As it turned out, our adult experiment in cohabitation lasted for over two years, until I moved in with my first husband. But the entire time Irmgard and I lived together, we had an actual line—drawn with a black Magic Marker—down the middle of her white kitchen counter, dividing my space from hers. Irmgard had marked the line, but not out of hostility. Rather, it symbolized my mother's insistence that we each create our own space within the home and respect the other's privacy.

"I don't believe in love anymore, Tina," she told me. "I only believe in respect. You can love someone and still be unkind to them or want them to change. But if you respect someone, you always have to show them that you accept them as they are."

Living with her, I learned another difference between the two. Love is messy, because it requires reciprocity, interaction, and flexible boundaries. Respect is pure and can be maintained even at a distance. Love draws others in. Respect keeps others out.

Irmgard allowed me into her life and heart more than she did with any other human being. But at some point she always drew a line.

IRMGARD WALKED. WHAT BEGAN as a routine to stay healthy gradually transformed into an addiction. While she worked full-time, she could be seen in rain, snow, sunshine, humidity, and bitter cold, striding along city sidewalks on the two-mile trip to the DuPont lab where she analyzed samples under an electron microscope. After her retirement, she chose the more scenic environs of the nearby former DuPont estates, with their manicured public gardens and well-groomed paths.

In the years I lived with her and afterward, my mother and I shared many strolls. Along various trails, past groves of cherry trees, fields of flowers, meadows, and ponds, we strode side by side. These outings took place through my master's degree coursework and internship, through my engagement, through my first marriage and divorce, and through my doctoral studies. I found them a calm and comforting counterpoint to the tumultuous vicissitudes of this period of my life.

Irmgard shattered the peace one cloudy, chill November day in 2003, as she and I ambled through some gardens discussing my upcoming PhD graduation. Furiously writing my dissertation nights and weekends, while working full-time and teaching an evening class, I worried I would not finish in time to walk with my classmates in the May 2004 commencement. The alternative was to take part in the December ceremony. As we talked about my graduation date, my mother's decision to die before she turned seventy obscured other thoughts in my mind. Her seventieth birthday fell in October 2004. I knew that if I graduated in May of that year, she would be there. If I graduated in December, according to her timetable, she wouldn't.

We had certainly discussed this dilemma before. In fact, all the conversations had followed a basic outline:

"You'll be there when I graduate, right?"

"Yes, I'll be there."

"If I work hard to get done in May, you won't do anything before then, right? Your plan is later in the year, right?"

"Don't worry, Tina. The date is not near your graduation."

"You promise you'll be there, don't you?"

"Yes, I promise."

"And you won't do it on a holiday, will you? I don't want to have to remember that you died on a holiday."

"No, Tina, it won't be on a holiday."

Our reiterations formed a clear pattern: my fear and her general evasiveness, my panic and her assurance. Whenever I brought up the subject, she tried to avoid talking about it. I always persisted. She thought discussing her death with me was "morbid," that "young people shouldn't have to think about old people dying." *But what am I supposed to do—pretend to have forgotten that you said you are going to kill yourself?*

And yet although the date remained an enigma, I knew with certainty that my mother wouldn't lie to me about her plans. Whether or not she would ultimately follow through, I couldn't say for sure. But she told me clearly she had a specific date in mind.

Consequently, if she promised she would participate in my graduation, then this was a pledge I could wrap around my aching heart. If she knew when she intended to end her life, she would also know what she would be able to do beforehand. My mother comforted and supported me, was my cheering section and my sounding board. I could not conceive of her setting out to mislead me.

Instead of doubting her veracity, I struggled at the time simply to imagine my life without my mother in it. During the most traumatic times of my life, I had always turned to Irmgard. Unwaveringly, she stood by my side and let me lean on her. In her quiet but steadfast manner, she steered me to rational courses of action. Who would guide me through the darkness that would surely overtake me when she was gone? How could I bear to let her go?

When I first moved in with her, she sensed my general unhappiness. By returning to Wilmington, I had left behind a car, an apartment, a job, and my closest friendships—in short, almost everything except my family. When I stepped off the airplane to begin our life together, my first words to her were, "I don't want to be here." She must have felt crushed by my insensitivity, having looked forward to her daughter's homecoming with such anticipation.

But she understood my feelings and concentrated on making our time together as meaningful as possible. Shortly after I arrived, she announced she would take a week's holiday from work and designated me the vacation planner. She would go anywhere I chose, only I had to be in charge of making the itinerary. As I pored over maps, then plotted out mileages and routes, made hotel reservations, and looked up restaurants, I experienced moments when memories of my former life began to fade into the background.

We toured New England together, walking through magical November morning snowfalls and visiting desolate historical sites, and I found myself pulled back more and more from the past into the present. We sat by cozy restaurant fireplaces every evening, rehashing the day's activities and planning upcoming adventures, and every day I felt slightly less bereft.

I had no idea that she had planned this all. Perhaps because of wisdom gained from her own experience of separating from her family, Irmgard had wanted to comfort and help me make peace with my decision to move back home. Knowing I felt buffeted by fate, she let me take control. Gradually I began to relax into the potential of a new life.

In 2003, long after those years we lived together, the thought of losing my mother increasingly terrified me. I feared change: a future of uncertainty, a future filled with regrets. The imagined hurt of losing her plagued me constantly. I dreaded that she and I, close as we were, would part with crucial words left unsaid, unspoken conflicts unresolved, unconscious worries unassuaged. I wanted to hang on to the life I knew and never face the grim anniversaries of "this time last year she was still . . ."

I had no religious or spiritual notions of what happens after death. I did not believe my mother's soul would outlast her physical being. But Irmgard, as areligious as I, repeatedly told me she believed that after her death a part of her spirit would live on inside me. Her favorite aunt, whom she loved dearly, had died when my mother was still in her teens. Irmgard explained that she could still have mental conversations with this aunt any time she wanted, because they had known each other so well. I would be able to do the same thing.

The idea appealed to me, and I fervently wanted to believe it. But it didn't ring true with anything in my own life experience and therefore brought me little comfort. How could I contemplate her spiritual presence in my future life when that future promised only the black hole of her absence?

As 2003 PROGRESSED AND the predicted date of my mother's death grew closer, my panic accelerated. Alone in bed from midnight to dawn, I frequently talked myself away from the edge of an abyss. I turned back and forth under the covers to move myself physically out of the way of the thoughts that followed me like balloons on a string. I sometimes toyed with the idea of giving in and throwing my psyche over the cliff of grief to see what happened. Imagine, I sometimes told myself, that she's gone. Imagine what that's like. Feel the pain.

But I couldn't.

The intensity of the pain defied my contemplation. To lose her seemed almost an annihilation of myself. And while I believed Irmgard completely capable of suicide, I couldn't perform emotional suicide in advance. *What would that prove, even if I were able to do it?* I thought. *If I do it once, jump over the edge to see what it will be like, what will prevent me from trying it again?*

My mother's dead. She's dead. Over and over and over again.

Even though I teetered on that edge, I did not lose my footing. But the more I thought things through, the more doomed I felt. It was a distant doom, to be sure, but it grew closer and more suffocating with each passing day.

EARLY ON, I HAD naturally attempted to talk my mother out of her plans. In long phone calls, weeping, I told her I would give up anything to spend more time with her. I said I would gladly sacrifice my own freedom to take care of her if she became incapacitated.

Irmgard flatly refused to change her mind. She didn't budge a micron. She would kill herself, and her mantra to me remained: "Tina, you can't change my mind, but the time is still so far in the future. Don't worry about all of this. I'll still be around for a long time. And now I don't want to talk about it anymore."

I believed if I actively opposed her, she would shut me completely out of this part of her life. *She's left me before. She can leave me again.* So I persuaded myself to uphold her decisions and declare her correct on all counts.

In doing that, I completely lost sight of myself.

Just as an abused child, in an effort to gain some control in a life of chaos and unpredictability, may eventually take on the role of abuser, I took on my mother's beliefs about the importance of respecting her wishes. I became her most ardent defender. Her will reshaped my reality. There soon came a point where I had difficulty picturing myself doing anything else but supporting her.

What began as a daughter's quest to understand the logic of her mother's decision to die ended in that daughter's devaluing her own grief. Although periodically overwhelmed with fear and sadness, I invariably tried to soothe myself by reminding myself that she was doing what was right for her. My showing respect and love for her (yes, I still believed in love) necessitated my supporting her and her position, without regard to the impact her death would have on me.

I knew what happened to someone who did not adopt this position and who instead tried to convince Irmgard of the error of her ways. She had told one of her close relatives vaguely of her plans many years before. In a more recent conversation with this relative, I mentioned the approaching date of Irmgard's planned death, believing he knew everything. My disclosure horrified him. From that point on he harangued my mother with letters and phone calls, believing he could persuade her to change her mind. Not surprisingly, she eventually wearied of his tirades and in the end lied to him outright. She told him the only thing he wanted to hear: that he had dissuaded her from killing herself. He believed her because he could not bear anything else. And after that she cut him out of her life.

I didn't want her to shun me. So in my words and in my actions my mother found nothing but support. *After all, we have always trusted each other*, I rationalized. *And she has always supported me.*

What I did not yet grasp was that Irmgard and I were both ignoring the obvious. First, she was not actually supporting me, at least not around the central issue of her intended demise. Instead, I was supporting her. And second, because she had told me of her plan and continued to discuss it with me, like it or not, she had intimately involved me in her decision and her process of carrying it out.

My feelings about this were as relevant and important as hers. They should not and could not be ignored.

Chapter 8

I Already Asked You

2003

G iven all I knew about my mother's intentions, why did I insist on repetitive, uncomfortable discussions about her death date? Why did her assurance that she would be present at my graduation not quell my anxieties? Did my worry focus on her presence or absence at this one event, or rather ooze throughout every crevice of our lives together? Or was something in the expression on her face during these conversations gnawing at me?

In late fall of 2003, we walked in the DuPont gardens again. As we headed across the parking area to our cars and discussed my May/December graduation quandary, I became aware of minor inconsistencies between her reassuring words and her nonchalant affect. Suddenly, apprehension overwhelmed me.

"Wait, Im. Before we go home, I have a favor to ask you," I said with my hands folded against the top of her open car door. "I'm sorry to bring this up again, but if I don't graduate in May next year, could you possibly promise to change your plans about your . . . well, you know, your death date, and be there at the ceremony in December?"

"Tina, do we have to talk about this again?" she asked wearily. Her voice had a slight edge of annoyance.

"Yes, I'm sorry. But I have to ask. Couldn't you just change your plans? December isn't far from your birthday in October. You wouldn't have to wait much. It would only be three or four months. Couldn't you just do this for me?"

My mother said nothing at first. She looked across the parking lot toward the slope leading to a private lake where, in winter, she and I sometimes crept to glide clandestinely across the inviting ice. "Okay, Tina," she replied, turning her eyes back to mine. "I'll be there."

Exultation and relief flooded my body. Feeling giddy, I was thankful to be leaning on the car door. "Im, thank you so much," I gushed. "I can't tell you how much pressure this takes off me. I'll do my best to finish the dissertation early, but I just don't know whether I'll get everything written in time to graduate in May."

She had acquiesced, and her face told me she didn't want to talk about this anymore. I simply grinned. As she climbed into her car, I reached out to hug her.

She hugged me stiffly in return.

"Tina, you don't have to thank me. It doesn't matter."

I removed my arms from around her. Cautiously, I held her gaze. "It doesn't *matter?*" And this time the realization came quickly. Once again, my mother had let something "slip," but this time the absolute callousness of her faux pas blew me away.

Aghast and outraged, I felt my heart constrict and my stomach heave. I knew the decision to change the date of her death mattered. There could only be one reason she said it didn't.

"You're lying to me," I breathed quietly. Then, fighting against the pressure in my chest I yelled, "You're lying to me! You're not going to be there for *either* graduation! You're planning to kill yourself *before* May, and you weren't going to tell me. You were just going to do it. And to me it was going to be a total surprise!"

"I'm sorry," she said without remorse. She held her head up proudly, defiantly. "I thought it would be best."

Blood drained from my face. Without asking, I walked to the passenger side of her car, got in, and slammed the door shut. I twisted in the seat to face her, angry tears flowing freely.

She sat behind the steering wheel with her hands in her lap, looking at me dry-eyed. "Tina, I did ask you, you know."

"You asked me? About what?" I snapped loudly, not caring whether anyone could hear us.

"About whether you would like me to have my final exit without saying goodbye."

"You never, ever asked me that!" I screamed. I felt sure beyond any doubt.

"Yes, I did. I remember clearly, because I did it deliberately. I wanted to know how you would feel about it. Don't you remember when I asked you about the Robert Redford movie *The Horse Whisperer*?"

"What does that movie have to do with anything?"

"Don't you remember that I asked you about whether you liked the ending? Robert Redford and his lover have a date to take one last horse ride, but his lover doesn't meet him. Instead, she drives off without saying goodbye. From the top of a hill he watches her car disappear. You said you liked the ending."

"*That* was supposed to be asking me how I felt about your killing yourself? You've got to be kidding! You asked me about a horse ride in a *movie*? It's just a movie! I can't believe you're saying this. How was I supposed to know you were asking me about *you*? And what does my liking the movie have to do with that anyway? I can't believe this!"

"I thought, since you liked that ending, where she broke a promise and didn't say goodbye, you wouldn't mind if I did the same thing."

An enormous boulder dropped into the ocean of my reality. The waves crashed against my consciousness.

I assailed her with questions. Why on earth had she hauled me through all this anticipatory grief only to end our relationship as though no preparation had taken place? If the date of her death were a complete unknown to me, her sudden demise would end up like any other suicide: an abrupt, shocking loss leaving only unanswered questions. I had always believed she dragged me through the years of foreknowledge to help us both prepare for the upcoming event, and to include as much consideration as possible for my future without her.

How on earth could she envision ending our relationship with a lie? The entirety of our mutual understanding was supposedly based on love, or at least mutual respect. If she told me one thing and deliberately did another, I would be left doubting the sincerity of not just this action but all of them. The shattered image of my mother would haunt me the rest of my life.

Obviously, I could not let our conversation end without a satisfactory resolution. We spent over an hour in the car that cloudy afternoon, hashing out the repercussions of her astonishing lack of empathy.

We reached only one solid conclusion: that she had made an error in judgment so momentous that she would consider, as a way of making amends to me, postponing her mystery death date for a year.

Consider. She made no promises.

Chapter 9

For Better or for Worse

2000

R on is my second husband. My first marriage failed dramatically, and sometimes I still blame myself for that. But I also believe it may very well have been doomed from day one.

My first husband and I had thoroughly enjoyed living together for almost a year before we tied the knot. Sam was a brown-haired, bearded official in local government in Delaware. At the time we met, I was a graduate student in social work. My brother introduced us, but only after a subsequent, serendipitous meeting did Sam and I decide we liked each other.

My father and I were walking through some newly opened park-land near Hans's house. As we strode along in conversation under the vine-covered cliffs, Sam whizzed by on his bicycle. I saw him and called out, "Hello!" He braked abruptly and got off, recognizing my father before he recognized me.

"It's nice to see you again, Sam," my father grinned. When he got no response, he continued. "Are you still working for the city?"

"Yes."

"Do you want to join us?"

Sam looked anxiously at his cleated bicycle shoes. "Well, I guess I could walk along for a bit."

He traipsed awkwardly at our side. The conversation progressed intermittently. My father grew bored and continued ahead at his longer-legged pace. Talking with me by myself, Sam eventually warmed up enough to ask me for a date. Over the course of a few months, we worked up to seeing each other regularly.

But from the start, I ignored signs that Sam was not the best choice for my life partner. When I met him, he was living in a bad part of Wilmington, so bad that even delivery people avoided it. Dealers sold drugs on the street corners. One morning we walked out of his home into a swarm of cops, guns drawn, raiding the row house two doors away. The trash-filled, hand-me-down jalopy Sam drove fit right in. His indoor décor also reflected the local environment, sporting touches such as exposed studs. Sam tore out many walls and ceilings in an ill-conceived home improvement effort, but after smashing the concrete to rubble with a sledgehammer, he lost interest. Jagged edges like broken teeth lined doorways. The bathtub sank into the floor, and from the toilet seat you could look through a hole into the basement. He lived in darkness, precipitated by the lack of adequate rewiring and perpetuated by a desire not to take stock of his actual circumstances. "I like candles," he evasively answered when I complained about having to negotiate my way in blackout conditions. Sam not only lived in a pseudo–war zone, he had also made his home into a bombed-out bunker.

In his house, there was only a hazy boundary between "out there" and "in here." And although I love wildlife, even I had to draw the line when feral creatures came inside and made themselves at home.

I woke up one night in his bedroom to hear a soft "tum, num, num" noise coming from the kitchen.

"Sam!" I shook him awake. "There's something in the kitchen. It might be a rat. It sounds like it's eating something."

Pause. "I don't hear anything. Go back to sleep."

"But Sam, how can you not hear that? Listen . . ."

"Num, num, tum."

"Just ignore it and go back to sleep."

"I'm not going to ignore it. We need to know what it is. We're going to have to do something about it in the morning."

"If you ignore it, it will be gone in the morning by itself."

"That's crazy. What if you have rats? And what if they come in here?" I got up hastily at the thought. The door between the bedroom and the kitchen had gone the way of the walls, so nothing separated the two spaces. I crept, ever so carefully, across the creaking floorboards toward the noise.

I stopped to listen. "Mum, tum, num." The sound came from the covered garbage can in the corner. With increasing apprehension, I carried over a wooden chair and found a broom. I didn't want to be too close to whatever was enjoying a meal in the can. I took the flashlight from the counter. The kitchen lacked light fixtures, making it a comfortable hangout for the nocturnal, furry set. I placed the chair next to the garbage can and climbed onto it, wondering whether this was a good idea. *What if it's a rat? What if it jumps?* I shined the flashlight beam onto the lid, and with the broom pole, I gingerly poked the cover open and illuminated the inside. There, reclining on a pile of refuse, lay a large opossum, bulging stomach exposed and front paws grasping a shred of sandwich. It looked up at me with a startled and slightly guilty gaze. "Caught me!" read the expression.

Compared to a rat, it seemed relatively cute and harmless, except that it stank and probably harbored fleas. For weeks it had been using Sam's overcoat, slung carelessly over a living room armchair, as a soft bed and his kitchen as its delicatessen. In Sam's house it led a life of luxury, especially with a human landlord who ignored its existence.

Despite Sam's protests that it was too much trouble, I declared that living with wildlife was unacceptable. The next day I borrowed my father's humane animal trap, and after a few frustrating mornings of waking to the sight of no peanut butter sandwich bait and no opossum, I finally caught the bugger. Sam and I relocated him to a park to lead a less cushy existence.

When I told my friends this story, they laughed. But their laughter felt slightly forced. From my accounts, Sam did not sound very attractive. And yet I felt drawn to him. Irmgard and I were still living together, which I enjoyed, but I was nonetheless ready to expand my circle of support. I had opened my heart to new adventures and had been passively looking for a romantic partner. I wasn't desperate, but I was certainly primed. Just at that time, Sam presented himself.

My concurrent studies in social work greatly increased his chances with me. Clinical social work students primarily want to be therapists, and the curriculum teaches them to see the promise in everyone. To give up and declare, "This person has no potential. He's not capable of change," in clinical social work is tantamount to an MBA student exclaiming, "We can never predict how economic markets work. So let's just give up on finance and management." If you think that way, you quickly learn you're in the wrong school. And I knew I wasn't in the wrong school.

Instead of examining the implications of his lifestyle choices and applying my conclusions to his potential behavior as a spouse, I saw Sam as someone whose life had room for improvement. To be honest, a lot of room. And when he explained he had recently initiated changes in his life, I believed him. I perceived someone like him, not quite my type, as a challenge. The challenge was not to completely refashion his personality, but rather to grow and expand my own horizons to be more accepting of who he was. For reasons pertaining to my prior relationships, I had decided I didn't want to be with someone who knew me so well he could guess my every move. Rather, I wanted someone who would make me more self-reliant.

My mother's exact plans were still unknown to me, but they also figured in my decisions. Because of them, I desired to become a stronger person in all my relationships. In addition, I thought that if my mother did follow through on her intentions, having a supportive partner by my side would help me weather the violent storm of her passing. To that end, I told Sam about my mother's suicide plans soon after we discussed marriage. Wanting him to know "what he was getting himself into," I also desperately wanted his comfort.

"Yes, Tina, I'll be there for you. You won't have to face it alone," he reassured me. In that, I heard what I wanted to hear. I ignored all the background noise.

For his part, Sam must have seen me as a breath of fresh air. I noticed things in him and believed things about him that, in hindsight, may not have been there. But Sam put on the best show he could for me, and the acting convinced me, because I wanted to believe. Unquestionably kind and extremely polite, he financed vacations financially far out of the reach of an unemployed grad student. He treated me with respect, admired my talents, and was generous about my flaws.

After a year of dating, we became engaged and decided to move in together as a prelude to marriage. I set one condition: that we not cohabitate in his dwelling. We would find a new place, I determined, in a neighborhood I approved of. By then I had convinced myself of the illusory idea that being able to leave his house meant Sam was capable of leaving his less attractive behaviors behind as well.

By then, I had invested a lot of time and emotion in the relationship, and I short-sightedly did not want to look too carefully at the mess I might be getting myself into. My mother wasn't getting any younger, either. When Sam and I announced our engagement, she was almost sixty-five years old. Seventy, her "expiration date," seemed just around the corner.

Sam and I regarded our year of living together in a rented condominium as a trial marriage. Since the experiment went well, we gathered our friends and family for a formal celebration of our union in the early summer of 2000. Neither of us could have predicted the disaster that would ensue immediately afterward. Instead, this forty-five-year-old husband and his thirty-five-year-old wife were almost cocky, naively sure that the practice cohabitation had provided a firm foundation on which to build a future together. But the evidence from Sam's past, evidence I had chosen to overlook, pointed clearly toward instability. And we newlyweds experienced not even a slight reprieve from disaster. Everything fell apart only one day after the wedding.

The afternoon following our marriage I came home to our bright, two-story condo. Wedding gifts we'd opened the night before and an empty bottle of champagne were strewn across the rug near the fireplace. I felt worn out from shuttling my friends around to our various morning-after receptions. My new husband lay on our cream-colored living room sofa, reading the newspaper with his feet propped up. I threw my car keys down onto the coffee table and fell to my knees in front of the couch. Putting my head on Sam's lap, I cried a few exhausted tears. I knew I was being overdramatic, but I felt sorry for myself. I yearned for a little, "There, there. Don't fret. Tomorrow we'll be off on our honeymoon, my love."

I waited for him to stroke my hair gently or wipe the tears from my cheek. Instead he did nothing. After a few moments, I glanced up. A look of life-changing horror passed over Sam's face. He let the newspaper fall and stared into my moist eyes. I could feel his entire body freeze, paralyzed by fear, and could sense what he thought: *What are you doing? Do you expect me to support you, to comfort you, to be responsible for you—from now on? Forever?* The weight of the idea crushed him.

"Sam, are you okay?" I asked.

"Uh-huh," he mumbled, his eyes darting away from mine.

"What's wrong? I can tell something is wrong."

"Nothing," he squeaked, reaching again for the newspaper.

"Don't read. I want to talk to you. What are you doing?"

"I'm reading." He propped the paper up between us.

My shock dissipated and was replaced by a flare of anger. "We're going to be on the plane tomorrow. I think you'll have enough time to read then." I stood, wiped my cheeks, turned my back on him, and marched upstairs. An hour later, when I had calmed down and nearly put the incident aside, I returned to the living room. Sam lay in exactly the same position, holding the newspaper. He had not turned the page.

My heart skipped a beat, and I realized something more troubling was wrong.

As inconceivable as it sounds, and although he would occasionally muster a bit of maturity and confidence afterward, the man I married had essentially disappeared. Subsequently, despite my reassurances about his personal inner strength and about my ability to hold my own in the world, the Sam I knew was gone. He morphed into a severely anxious, unimaginably insecure person with whom I felt no connection whatsoever. I had glimpsed parts of this person before the marriage: Sam's underlying anxieties had certainly been behind the creation of his disastrous living space, for example. But

I had never thought of living with that part of him. I concentrated on ignoring it. In our own ways, Sam and I had each been good at self-deception.

We were locked into a two-week honeymoon on the island of Bermuda, which I had been looking forward to with immense anticipation. But as my mother and my friends saw us off at the airport gate in Philadelphia, a sudden feeling of dread washed over me, and I did not want to go.

Sure enough, among the pastel houses and pink sands, we lived a nightmare. With no way off the island, no individual transportation, and no possibility of separate rooms, Sam and I were essentially sharing a prison cell fashioned from the walls of his uncontrolled fears. Outside the sun shone, the birds called, the ocean waves glided back and forth across the beach. Inside, we were trapped in hell.

Rapidly, Sam's inner strength and personality disintegrated. He floundered under the weight of even the smallest decision, terrified that he would make the "wrong" choice. He became almost immobilized, to the point that he had to mimic my actions in order to retain the semblance of living. He followed me everywhere and did everything I did, becoming my perverse shadow. Only after I picked up my fork at the dinner table, did he. Only when I stabbed a piece of food and brought it to my mouth, did he. If I caught on to his behavior and suddenly dropped my fork back onto the plate, food untouched . . . so did he. And if I addressed directly the farce we were acting out or tried to counsel him through what I took at first to be transitory, post-wedding jitters, he retreated into a silent, hardened shell.

Only later would I draw coherent conclusions about what had happened. For Sam, marriage represented an overwhelming responsibility. The marriage took on hidden, destructive meanings that shattered our otherwise reasonably strong, if shakily grounded, relationship. Sam was equally surprised by what lurked beneath the surface of his consciousness. Because he had been unknowingly playing a part, he had not been aware of the implications our union held for him, or for us.

By the time we returned to the States, I had made my own warped peace with the insane situation. My behavior shocked my mother severely when she picked us up at the airport. In just two weeks, the relationship between her daughter and her new son-in-law had disintegrated from one of equals to that of an overbearing mother with a small child. Ten years Sam's junior, I had nevertheless taken to ordering him around: "Pick that up. Come here. Sit down." He obsequiously complied with these direct commands, as though knowing how to act gave him some measure of comfort in his misery. To me, taking charge felt like the only way I could get him to do anything. But it did not set a good tone for the time to come.

Excruciating months passed, as he and I tried everything I could think of to get back to where we had been before that fateful day in May—therapy, anti-anxiety medication, support groups, antidepressants, and talk after talk after tearful midnight talk. Nothing worked long or well enough. Eventually he and I would return to the honeymoon dynamic that repeated the pattern of his youth. In his mind, his parents haunted and berated him. He became the terrified child. And I became the domineering figure forcing him to relive his past.

By some fluke of psychological functioning, Sam still managed to hold down a full-time job despite all his personality disturbances. His coworkers noticed he was not on an even keel, but through various mental contortions, he performed just well enough not to get fired.

One afternoon, when I had reached yet another breaking point, I telephoned him at work. I asked that he shut his office door and simply listen. I had begun seeing a therapist regularly, to understand my responsibility for the horrific dynamics that were unfolding. But I felt beleaguered by the immensity of his resistance to change. "Sam, you were someone else before," I told him. "Reach into yourself and find that person again, or I don't think I can continue in this marriage." My insides shook with fear in anticipation of how he would react.

"Okay, Tina, I'll do my best," was his uncharacteristic response. Even in the tone of his voice I could discern a small difference. I began to have hope.

Miraculously, the Sam I met at the front door that evening was the old Sam. Before he even took off his coat, I could see the change in his expression and in his movements. He had self-assurance again, and a personality independent of mine. He was decisive and friendly, funny and kind, thoughtful and assertive. He swung his overcoat flamboyantly off his shoulders, as though he were removing his cares, and hung it in the hallway closet. I watched intently for a sign of collapse. Sam instead took me into his arms.

"You seem great," I whispered.

"I feel fine," he intoned in his confident baritone. "I feel like a new person. I think I just needed to pull myself together."

"I'm so glad you're back," I said, nuzzling against his neck, feeling warm for the first time in weeks. "I didn't know what I was going to do if . . ."

Sam cut me off. "Don't worry. It's over now."

We did not discuss the change much, afraid that in its fragile state it would shatter. Instead, it crumbled slowly. Within weeks the crippling anxiety returned. And I began to recognize that this, not his previous self, represented the true essence of his personality.

Although my family and friends realized something was amiss, I hid the depths of my desolation from them for as long as I could. *How can I explain things when I hardly understand them myself*, I thought. *And what does it say about me that I chose to ignore the warning signals I saw early on?*

I made excuses for Sam with my father, which Hans seemed to believe. But my relationship with my mother suffered, because she, with her mantra of respect, began to demur at coming over to our house or spending time with me when Sam might be present. She could not tolerate seeing me treat someone else with such disregard. Because of that, living with Sam became even more disturbing for me. I struggled with the knowledge that, if I stayed with him and Irmgard killed herself, dealing with Sam's reaction and his needs would make working through my own grief exponentially more demanding.

SAM HAD OBVIOUSLY SUFFERED when he was young. Even the most rudimentary understanding of emotional development would indicate there was a childhood event or series of events that had created this shut-down version of him.

He had grown up with an alcoholic father. But his mother made the stronger impression on everyone who met his parents. From what I saw, Sam's mother could be astoundingly harsh and overbearing, to the point of frightening even adults. She reacted unkindly to criticism, and no one I knew opposed her wishes. I could only imagine what it was like to grow up under such an unforgiving rule.

Of course, I only knew Sam's mother as a seventy-something matriarch, but even at that age she still wielded an emotional iron fist over her children. One Christmas, during the family's traditional three-day holiday extravaganza, I invited all Sam's siblings and their spouses over to our home. I thought it would be relaxing for us to get together for a few hours, sans kids and sans parents. Sam's mother had a fit. Such insubordination—having a party to which she was deliberately uninvited—had never occurred in her family. She called us nine times that morning, hardly able to contain her frustration and resentment. She invented myriad reasons why this gathering was "a disastrous idea" and threatened to obstruct it. It turned out to be the only instance in my brief relationship with most of my sisters- and brothers-in-law that I heard all of them talk about growing up emotionally isolated from their parents and, as they each cautiously confessed, from each other.

But over time I became less and less interested in unearthing the origins of Sam's behavior. Instead, I became more and more focused on how to get out of the marriage.

Eventually, I told everyone about my suffering. And when I expressed my ambivalence about leaving or staying, a wise friend counseled me, "Don't worry. When the pain gets to be too much, you'll leave him."

It turned out I could take more pain than I gave myself credit for.

Our life together was absolutely wretched, but letting go of the possibility of Sam's transformation and of my faith in my ability to choose a good partner seemed to me, for a long while, even worse. And as I struggled to make a decision, Sam dug his head even further into the sand. For him, anything other than emotional paralysis seemed like purgatory.

At the end, by all measures our marriage was a farce. No physical intimacy, no emotional connection. I shudder when I think of the fights our neighbors must have heard—my side of the fights, that is. Sam hardly ever spoke during them or raised his voice. At the first hint of anger, he retreated immediately into silence and then tears. My efforts to provoke any kind of reaction escalated to mortifying proportions. I threw books, china, even furniture. I screamed at the top of my lungs. I called him things one should never say within earshot of anyone who understands English.

Torn between the hell of living together and the fear of facing our own failures, we both suffered through two trial separations. In the end, however, the pain did become too much to bear. One morning my therapist asked me, "Tina, do you want to live with Sam? Not the Sam he used to be. Not the Sam you think he can be. Just Sam, as he is now." The stronger half of me finally said no.

That afternoon, at the end of the summer of 2002, Sam and I talked in our sunlit bedroom. He sat in the armchair by the bed and I knelt on the floor, in an attempt to look directly into his eyes. I took his hands in mine. I told him that we had both tried for a long time to fix what was broken in our relationship, but that nothing had worked, and nothing was going to work. I told him I could do nothing else. Then I asked him to leave.

He agreed, without resistance or regret.

Our divorce was final in March of the following year, ending one of the bleakest and most difficult chapters of my life to that point.

And yet I would face much worse in the all-too-near future.

Chapter 10

Mondays

2004

After our argument at the DuPont gardens, Irmgard did elect to postpone her theoretical date. I took this as a sign of respect for me and as perhaps the smallest crack in her resolve to exclude my feelings from her process.

In the months following that conversation, I came to know the details of her plans bit by bit. Much as a parent cautions a child not to bite off more than she can chew, my mother always met my requests for details with, "Do you *really* want to know?" Honestly, many times I didn't. I knew enough. I knew I had a year.

Irmgard did attend my graduation ceremony, which took place in May 2004 after all. On that day, as on most days then, I thought briefly of my mother's impending death, but these thoughts by no means dominated. By that time, I excelled at compartmentalizing my feelings about losing my mother. Instead I remember beautiful sunshine and an increasingly warm tent, loud clapping and cheers as I walked across the stage, and my high school–age nephews jokingly wearing my comical doctoral cap at the reception.

Nevertheless, as the end of summer approached, the countdown to Irmgard's planned date began in earnest. It affected me immensely. In incremental fragments I learned that her suicide was arranged for 2005, then that it would take place in the first half of that year. Eventually she narrowed it down to February.

USUALLY, THE PART OF me that feared my mother's death struggled in isolation. But as 2004 progressed, I told a number of friends the truth about my mother and her plans. I could no longer keep this traumatic secret to myself. The confession often simply burst out of me. Topics of conversation just didn't work themselves around to death all that often, and I couldn't think of a graceful segue to saying, "My mother's planning to kill herself in a few months."

Yet for all the inelegance of my announcement, my friends reacted kindly. Although they may have felt they had no choice. I would not have responded well to someone openly criticizing my mother and her plans. My mother gave me no alternative but to accept her decision. I needed my friends to accept it too, if they were going to be my companions and support me through the coming months. In retrospect, I constructed the same dynamic my mother forced on me: accept or be shut out.

My brother and father, however, felt no such obligation. Neither had swallowed my mother's viewpoint hook, line, and sinker. Consequently, neither was able to have meaningful conversations with her about the subject. She closed herself to them. But they also remained more in touch with their own emotional reactions to her decision.

Warner sometimes talked with me about his struggles with our mother. Although I didn't share all his opinions, they struck a chord. His reactions vacillated between denial and anger, and he expressed each vehemently within our small family. Faith in the idea that she would never go through with it would tide him over for a few weeks, and then his confidence would crack. During those moments stronger emotions seeped out—rage; justifiable indignation at the idea; righteous resentment about her selfishness; and deep sadness. "I'll never have anything to do with her if she goes through with it," may seem like a ridiculously illogical statement, but a piece of me resonated with what he meant.

Hans did not have much contact with Irmgard, so his conversations about the matter took place mostly with Warner and with me. Above all, Hans was scared. The idea of his children losing their mother prematurely brought up painful memories of his own losses. Hans supported me, but in his heart he never wanted to believe Irmgard would really carry out her plan.

From my perspective at that time, children with parents suffering from cancer, Alzheimer's, or other drawn-out diseases had a luxury denied me: the ability to talk openly about their situation. "How's your mom doing today?" acquaintances could ask them. Or "How are you holding up?" These might not always be the most welcome questions, but I longed for people to ask how I was, to give me some sympathy, to distract me for a while. I had been living at the opposite end of the empathy spectrum. From the self-induced solitude of my vantage point, I experienced sadness, fear, anger, and abandonment in a relative vacuum. My need for support grew in inverse proportion to the time I had left with Irmgard. Yet I could not reach out beyond my small circle of friends, because I could not risk encountering someone who would smash my façade, someone who would bring me face to face with the truth that Irmgard's decision was really not okay with me, and that I needed her to know this.

In addition, I lacked the wishful anticipation that people in difficult situations often have—the sense that no matter how wild or medically unjustified the expectation, death can be postponed or a miracle recovery can be achieved. That with a new treatment or medicine or with the strongest optimistic outlook anything is possible. Family members of dying loved ones can cling to hope to stave off a sense of overwhelming doom.

Instead, the doom enveloped me.

But I was never completely alone. My best friend, Lucy, had been aware of the truth for many years. She and I had known each other since we were babies, when our German-immigrant, first-time mothers sought solace and panicked advice from each other about raising toddlers. Once they put us together, we became inseparable, two female infants united against our two brothers and the world. When she was five, Lucy's family moved back to West Germany, but we managed to remain in touch. Summer visits to my relatives across the ocean invariably included spending days or weeks with Lucy's family, and she came to the States with her family on holiday as well. Over the years, she and I built almost as many memories together as we would have accumulated had we lived closer together. Perhaps because our visits were so brief, we never fought, and we never tired of each other's company. On the beach or on the playground, in the pool having underwater tea parties or in the attic trying on her grandmother's nineteenth-century clothing, Lucy and I were inseparable.

On several occasions, she attended summer camp with me in Pennsylvania. We savored the unlimited hours we could spend together, swimming, playing sports, or making crafts. But our concentration on having fun together left little time to interact with other campers or to make new friends. Even the counselors tended to think of us as interchangeable. So on Awards Night the first year, Lucy sat gloomily in the buggy darkness around the campfire, trying not to let the golden light shine on her nervous face. Sitting beside me, she looked fixedly down at the ground. As counselors called camper after camper to the fore to proudly receive an award for "Best Kickball First Baseman" or "Dirtiest T-Shirt," Lucy crouched lower and lower.

"Tina," she pulled at my arm, "let's go."

"Why?" I whispered, confused.

"This isn't any fun. I'm never going to get anything. Nobody knows me."

I looked down at my own red Magic Marker award, scrawled onto a white cardboard cutout, and wondered for the first time about her. I was certain she would not be forgotten, but suddenly put on the spot, I could not come up with reassuring examples of her summer achievements that would be worthy of public recognition.

"And now . . . Lucy!" a counselor's voice boomed through the smoky air, interrupting our conversation. "Lucy?" she called again.

"Hey, that's you," I nudged her.

She rose slowly, and I could see her expression wavering between excitement and disbelief. She stepped over other children's outstretched, mosquito-bitten legs on her way around the campfire. As she stood in front of the counselor, I held my breath.

"When we look for Lucy," the young woman announced, "we've learned all we have to do is look for Tina. Lucy will be close by. So tonight, Lucy, we present you with the 'With Tina' award!"

The clapping rang in my ears, and across the fire, Lucy sought out my eyes, her face flushed with pride. They had managed to pinpoint the most wonderful achievement of our summer after all.

Years later, we remain close. Although we live on opposite sides of the country, we have regular phone dates, and we can easily talk for hours at a stretch. We began this ritual soon after she moved to California in 1996, and it became one of the linchpins of my existence. A week did not quite seem real until I had rehashed every important event with her.

And so, throughout the years my mother planned her demise, Lucy walked beside me on whatever path I chose to follow. I don't even remember when I first broached the subject with her, but I do remember she was not surprised by Irmgard's choice. She had known my mother almost as long as I had, and she knew that what my mother decided, my mother usually did.

In addition to Lucy, I relied upon Hans. Despite his desire to ignore Irmgard's plans, he remained someone I could turn to, a supportive shoulder, literally and figuratively. More than once I called him in tears from my condo and he responded immediately, "Should I come over?" My answer was always "Yes." When he walked through the door, I fell into his arms and he simply held me, offering the comfort of his presence instead of his words. Nevertheless, all our interactions around the subject of Irmgard ended with his question, "You don't really think that she is going to do it, do you?"

What could I say except, "I don't want her to, but I think she will."

Immediately defeated, he would admit, "Yes, I guess it's possible. I just hate to see you suffering so much."

"It's okay, Hans." I would say. "I appreciate your being here. It is hard, but I will make it. Somehow."

THROUGH ALL OF THIS, I increasingly felt a desire for the input of a neutral professional. I had gone to a therapist during my divorce and found her very helpful. Now, on the brink of another major life event, I went to see Sarah again.

My seeking outside help displeased my mother. She did not like to discuss her plans at length with me or anyone else. She reacted coldly every time I mentioned I had told one of my friends, and she felt even more uncomfortable that I was sharing information about it once a week with "a stranger."

Part of me also dreaded the weekly Monday evening appointments with Sarah. But mostly I needed one environment in which I, not Irmgard, was the center of attention with regard to this nightmare.

Irmgard had a different reason to dread my sessions, because through them I learned to express my pain. Sitting in the dark parking lot outside Sarah's office every Monday, I called Irmgard on my cell phone. Sometimes in tears, sometimes in anger, I left a message on her answering machine. Irmgard never answered the phone, because she always wanted time to digest the task I set before us. Generally, I asked her to talk about a very specific reaction or thought that had emerged during therapy. In that fashion, like it or not, my mother became a participant in the emotional work that therapy showed me I had to do.

Therapy task number one: Have Tina acknowledge her own feelings about her mother's potential death.

"Feelings? What feelings? I'm fine with it," was my oh-so-resilient refrain, so well rehearsed that I never thought to question its authenticity. I spent countless hours with Sarah attempting to find out just what my emotions were.

People whose loved ones are dying of natural or traumatic causes are often accused of being in denial of death. Actually, denial can be a very helpful and protective psychological mechanism. It is often part of the grieving process and can begin before the actual loss occurs. But my circumstances disallowed that comfortable if temporary respite from reality.

A physician friend found my description of anticipatory sadness out of place. I had blurred the true context by telling him my mother was dying of cancer, and he admitted he had never encountered a person who accepted the finality of such a diagnosis and its consequences as completely as I did. I did not rail against the probable outcome or hold out even the smallest hope for a recovery or a brief remission. Why, he wondered, were my reactions so strangely counterintuitive?

Of course, they were counterintuitive in the context of cancer, but this wasn't cancer. This wasn't any type of disease. This was premeditated, methodical, and seemingly inescapable suicide.

I FELT BOUND TO certain conditions in order to continue my relationship with Irmgard during that time. Feeling she gave me no choice, I adopted the impartial and principled perspective that she was exercising her prerogative to end her own life. Consequently, I became her defender. I assigned myself the role of shielding my mother from all attackers. And in that role my primary nemesis was me.

Who had more to lose than I from her death? Consequently, from whose emotions did I face the most devastating attack? It turned out to be my own.

I took whatever escape route I could get. I denied my feelings about everything hurtling toward me.

Sarah regularly asked, "How do you feel about all of this?"

I always met this question with the same response: "I'm sad, but I know she has the right to do this if she really wants to." That she had the right to do this was, of course, not the point.

I FIRST REJECTED MY own emotions and then had those same emotions careen out of control.

Nothing in the current literature suggests that the experience of grief takes place in the form of a one-way ladder—that once you've left one rung, you can never revisit it, or that the process is in any way locked into a forward gear. Instead, contemporary thinking on grief might envision the emotional reactions as intersecting circles. Everyone who has experienced loss knows it's quite possible to inhabit more than one circle at the same time, or to move through a number of them in rapid succession. Typically, people perceive the pain associated with bereavement as messy rather than neatly defined.

Given the almost complete lack of hope I had for my mother's survival past February, I found myself wading quite far into dark waters well in advance of the actual loss. In this I was not unique. Any impending loss can conjure many anticipatory reactions. I simply had the opportunity to indulge in almost two decades of them.

When you think about it, all of us could continually be wallowing in anticipatory grief. All we have to do is look around at anyone or anything we are attached to. Instead of concentrating on this present moment, we can focus on the time when that person or thing will no longer be around. The cat crouched here on the desk beside my computer—well, her days are numbered. Ron downstairs writing? He can eat all the vegetables I feed him and bike all over creation, and I'll still probably outlive him by twenty years. It's a rather depressing pastime, this divestiture of the beloved, if you start thinking about it too much.

This explains why I didn't spend all my time dwelling on my mother's upcoming departure. Death is part of life. Although we all know this, most of us spend more time with the daily process of living at the center of our attention. The only difference in my situation was that the loss of my mother seemed not only inevitable but, barring a freak accident or illness on her part, also completely predictable.

Because of this unwelcome clairvoyance, I had accumulated a closetful of emotional reactions to the situation over many years. Unfortunately, my reactions mostly took place without my acknowledgment, so when I finally released my sadness and anger, their intensity astonished me. In Sarah's lamp-lit office, freed by roleplaying and by being left alone to cry unashamedly, I slowly and excruciatingly uncovered feelings I had long been defending myself against. Before, I had only been looking at my mother. With Sarah's help I now turned my view inward to regard a screaming part of myself jailed in a corner of my soul. Letting that grief-ridden woman out of her cell took no small measure of courage, for I was not at all familiar with her hair-tearing, wailing ways. And I wasn't quite sure how she would react to freedom.

You're completely irrational, I told this painful revelation of my emotional self. *And you're not really a part of me. I don't want to deal with your rebelliousness. I'm perfectly happy with my rational approach to what's happening. I don't want to spend my days and nights crying, especially about something that hasn't even happened yet. Basically*, I told that wild woman inside my heart, *I would like to get through all this without having to face my grief. So I'd thank you very much to stay where you are.*

Of course, had those been my true thoughts, I would not have taken myself to therapy in the first place. I could not completely ignore the irony of the situation.

And yet learning that acknowledging my own sadness did not merely require that I face my own grief shocked me. The wild woman wasn't just wild with sorrow. She was also hopping mad. And at me, of all people!

Therapy task number two: Acknowledge your anger.

Okay, the wild woman yelled in my head, *so Irmgard said you had to accept her position or be booted out of her inner circle of friends. But you just stood there and took it! You never bothered to stand up for yourself and say, "Hey, I'm your daughter, and what you're doing is selfish. I support your right to be selfish, but let's face it: killing yourself hurts me. It's high time you acknowledge that." Noooo, you didn't want to rock the boat! Your mother's precious feelings were more important than your own. You say you have this great relationship with her, but can you really call it a relationship if she's calling all the shots?*

Of course, the wild woman knew exactly how to pull apart my charade. In the end, battered, I decided to open the cage carefully and let her out. On probation. Just to see what happened. As thanks, she ripped the door off its hinges and assailed me and my mother with a vengeance.

After I set her free, I took up sobbing as a serious hobby. I definitely improved my weeping skills on Monday nights, driving back home after therapy. Once I even turned on the windshield wipers, mistaking the overflowing water in my eyes for rain. I cried at work, at home, upon hearing my mother's favorite music in yoga class, and when picking out birthday cards in the grocery store.

Only I didn't cry in my mother's presence. I couldn't bring myself to open up to her. I still feared she would take this as a sign of disapproval. While I did indeed disapprove, I did not trust her not to exclude me from her life entirely.

To a disconcerting degree, and not surprisingly, patterns forged during my childhood influenced my adult behavior. The abandoned child of a divorce could not face another abandonment. Especially because the future offered no hope for reconciliation.

So I didn't let my mother see my tears. But over the course of numerous conversations, the wild woman and I cautiously challenged her to recognize my role in our symbiotic drama. Irmgard reacted coolly at first, as if she were unable to see how the two of us could reach an understanding. We had both become so used to my being her unwavering supporter that injecting my own, sometimes contrary notions into our relationship seemed completely out of place.

Neither of us knew quite what to do with the fact that I didn't want her to kill herself. For so many years we had equated my support for her right to die with complete acquiescence to her desires. My newly unleashed anger and defiance scared both of us.

In truth, I still clung to my desire for a mother figure, one who would put all my needs above her own. And some part of her still desired a daughter who would do her bidding without question. In therapy I came to realize the only way for us to move along together in this, for me to stand by her side as an adult, as a friend, and as a companion on her journey, was for me to no longer act as her clone. And for her not to need me to.

Eventually, I told her everything I was feeling, which went something along the lines of: "I don't want you to die, ever. And given that you have to die at some point, I don't want it to be anytime soon. Your killing yourself is a selfish act. It will hurt me a great deal, and you say you are going to do it anyway.

"But don't ever say that you're doing it 'for your children,' because that is an utter lie. You are doing it against your children's wishes. You're doing it because it's right for you. But that doesn't make it right for anyone else. What you are going to do will rip each of your children apart. And until you acknowledge the pain that you are inflicting on others because of your selfish desires, you and I are not going to be able to move honestly through this process.

"My feelings are different from my rational thoughts. I can respect your right to make this choice without agreeing with the choice. I will never agree with this choice. But I think you can let my pain become part of your experience without becoming overwhelmed with the fear that it will change your mind."

Chapter 11

A Piece of Work

2004

E ntangled in the web of the present, it is often difficult to see that the threads now binding us extend far back into the past. That a current crisis is inextricably connected to faint glimmers of experiences from long ago. That love in the present may be shaped by how love was given and received before.

I found this to be the case with Irmgard.

"Excuse me for saying this, honey, but I just have to tell you that your mother is a piece of work!" Patsy shouted into the telephone receiver.

This outburst occurred not long after I learned of Irmgard's proposed February 2005 end date, which I had shared with my close friend. Patsy's vehemence left me speechless. While I waited in shocked silence for her to continue, I heard her take a deep breath.

She then continued more quietly. "I'm sorry, Tina, to say something like that about your mother, I truly am. You know I've met your mother, and she seems very nice. She really seems very kind. But I've just been thinking about all you're going through and I had to pick up the phone and call.

"Actually, I should be talking with your mother, not with you. I want to ask her how she can put her daughter through this. Telling you she's going to kill herself. And telling you years in advance, so that you'd have this hanging over your head for decades. What in God's name was she thinking?

"Forgive me, but if she wants to kill herself, she should do it on the sly, like normal people, and just leave you a long note explaining everything. Why all this drama ahead of time? Why does she need to be the center of attention for so long? Who's she trying to get back at? Because she's certainly not paying any attention to you or *your* feelings."

Patsy's outrage confused me. Nevertheless, therapy had taught me to know better than to tumble into an automatic defense of my mother. And yet I heard myself say, "I know it can seem that way, Patsy. And I don't mind your saying these things. But actually, I think what my mother's planning to do can be seen as a very logical decision . . ."

"*Logical!?*" she interrupted. "What's logical about telling your daughter you're planning to die? Not planning to die tomorrow, but planning to die *decades* from now! Tomorrow, I could maybe still understand." Patsy paused to consider. "Maybe I could even understand six months from now, or a year. That's what some people with cancer get. But nobody gets a twenty-year warning. Hell, we could all have twenty-year warnings. We just don't know about them. That's the whole point. We keep on living and laughing *because we don't know!*" Her voice abruptly softened and she asked, "How on earth have you held yourself together, child?"

Tears welled up in my eyes, and for a moment I could not answer. Finally, I choked out, "I don't know. I guess I just thought this was the way things had to be. So I dealt with it."

REMARKABLY, BEFORE HAVING IT pointed out to me, I never considered that my mother's plans for death could have been separated from her choosing to tell me about them. That Irmgard could have contemplated exactly the same ideas but let me in on her secret differently. That she could have simply gone through with the act and left me a note, or only given me a year's warning.

And if telling me had been a matter of choice, conscious or otherwise, then why not refrain?

Kind and caring mother though she was, a latent psychological desire also motivated her actions. But a desire for what? Payback? Certainly not payback for something *I* had done to her. But perhaps payback for something that had happened in her childhood?

When Irmgard received the phone call telling her that her

mother had died, she immediately called me. I was in high school and cried when I heard the news. I had spent weeks with my grandparents in Germany during summer vacations, and although my grandmother could be demanding, I had learned how to burrow my way into her heart. I brought baskets of gooseberries in from her backyard fruit plots, set the lunch table before I was asked, and coaxed her onto the garden swing, pushing her higher and higher, until she laughed uncontrollably as her apron flew over her head. In turn she had rewarded me with outpourings of easy, warm intimacy.

I knew my mother had a conflicted relationship with my grandmother, that Irmgard could talk of happy times with her mother one minute and disparage her the next. But her not wanting to attend the funeral surprised me.

"She died for me a long time ago, Tina," Irmgard said. "You can go if you want to, but I don't have any reason to. I already said my goodbyes."

I went to the funeral alone, but my mother's inconsistencies troubled me. Her attitude toward her mother was only one of many examples. Irmgard maintained an adamant stance that nothing from her past affected her anymore, but at the same time German history obsessed her. She had strained and at the same time needy relationships with her brothers. In her words she dismissed all attachments to her childhood, but she showed a simultaneous sentimentality toward letters, photos, and mementos. Could it be that these contradictory impulses signified something, or many things, that could not be named? Had she shoved people or events into a closet in her mind and locked the door forever as a way to protect herself?

It was possible, perhaps even probable. Something had been inflicted on Irmgard to make her punish the person who loved her most. How deeply she must have been hurt as a child to be able to justify hurting me in a strange form of revenge, hoping to attain a kind of quid pro quo, however misdirected and unconscious.

Or was she satisfying a deep-seated craving for attention by telling me of her plans so early? Did she need to guarantee always being center stage in my relationship with her?

She certainly achieved that. Because of her announcement, I

made life decisions that revolved around her. I moved back to Wilmington and into her condo partially—mainly—because I believed our time together was limited. All her pooh-poohing of my wanting to discuss her decision with her, all her declarations that I made "too big a deal of this" in reality represented earsplitting cries to make a big deal of it. To pay attention. To notice.

Everyone knows Andy Warhol's remark that we all get our fifteen minutes of fame. But with me Irmgard stretched her fifteen minutes to more than fifteen years.

And, ironically, she didn't have to do it. Since my childhood, she had shown me tremendous affection, and I returned it multifold. Apart from our fleeting, temperamental blowups, I enjoyed her company and sought it out. On parents weekend at my New England college, for all four years I invited only my mother. She slept in my dorm room bed while I slept in a sleeping bag on the floor. I dragged her around campus and proudly introduced her to my friends and professors. We hiked in the nearby mountains together and dined at eclectic restaurants, where I treated her with money I had scrimped together from my campus job.

So after all that, why on earth did she need more of my attention? Or could it have been a test?

Despite my boundless outpouring of caring, the usually confident Irmgard sometimes did not believe I truly loved her. She would occasionally blindside me by coldly accusing me of the most appalling lack of regard. If I professed having a new love in my life, having opened my heart to someone else, eventually she would use that as an excuse to pull away from me. Instead of being happy for me, she felt threatened, as though she believed my love existed only in limited supply and her share would diminish.

Before my engagement to Sam, Irmgard and I had begun to plan a brief vacation to the beach. We had both been looking forward to it. I had gathered information about possible hotels and finalized our dates for travel when, suddenly one evening, she called me into her bedroom and announced, "Tina, you weren't engaged when we started making these plans, but you're engaged now. You should go to the beach with Sam, not me. You don't want to go with your mother. You want to go with your fiancé."

Whoa. Hold on! Who doesn't want to go with whom here? The next hours shocked me because, no matter what I said, she held on to that line: "You don't want to go with your old mother. You are young. I know you really want to go with a young person." Never mind that she and I had thoroughly enjoyed a similar trip the previous year. That Sam and I had vacations planned of our own. That her age or my marital status had no impact on my thinking at all. She would simply not believe I wanted to go with her.

Obviously, her part of the conversation was not at all about me. She was projecting from her past. I realized this even at the time, and it frightened me. I felt as if my mother had lost her grasp of reality and had sunk into a deep hole beyond my understanding. And although we did end up taking the vacation together, I never forgot that night.

PAYBACK? ATTENTION SEEKING? TESTING? It could have been all of these. And they are not all the possibilities. Some people might say Irmgard's need to tell me of her suicide plans so far in advance had to do with darker motives—that my mother had a sadistic streak; that she deliberately hurt me because I symbolized someone else who had purposely hurt her.

This is possible.

I never directly questioned her motives for telling me years ahead of time. For too long and in too many ways I had succumbed to Irmgard's mantra: my way or the highway. And because I loved her and did not want to lose her, I had years ago chosen to do things her way. At the time and for a long time afterward, it did not even feel like a choice. I felt I had no other option. I couldn't even contemplate options. She may have felt powerless at some point in her past, but now, in regard to her plans, she had control.

I heard Patsy make her point, but by the time she expressed it to me, it was too late. I couldn't take it in. By that juncture, as much as I might learn to express my feelings, in some ways I could hold no other perspective than my mother's. Too isolated and bound up in the present, I could not see Irmgard's actions with any objectivity. To be with Irmgard, I had to lose part of myself.

I could look deeply into my torturer's eyes. But I could not feel pain.

Worse, I was learning to become a torturer myself.

Chapter 12

Travels

2004

My mother never attended any therapy sessions with me. Sarah and I worked through my resistance to introspection and Irmgard's resistance to acceptance alone. But the process continued outside the sessions, and this required Irmgard to be ready to engage in meaningful conversation with me followed by meaningful action.

Irmgard's willingness to change her default stance—"Let's not talk about my death"—spoke volumes about her feelings for me. I would leave a message on her answering machine about a task I determined we needed to tackle; she would call me back the next day, ready to discuss it.

For example, I realized it would comfort me to eliminate some of the mystery around her plans. Without any grounding, I was beginning to visualize the most gruesome scenarios: shooting; drowning; electrocution; hanging. As my hypothetical list became longer and longer, I grew more and more fearful.

"I need to know how you're going to do it," I told her machine bluntly one Monday evening. When we met to talk Thursday afternoon, Irmgard showed signs of great hesitation.

"Tina," she sighed, "do you really want to know *that?*"

"If I don't know, I'll continue to have these awful nightmares. Can you imagine what this is like for me? It's like knowing you have cancer but not knowing what kind of cancer. I think of you dying in the most horrible ways."

"I guess I don't really know what you're going through." We

gazed at each other. We didn't speak. Then she placed her hand over mine and rose from the oval table in her living room where we were sitting.

"Wait here," she said.

I looked around the room, taking in the white wall, white ceiling, many windows, minimal furniture, and no clutter. *I can't see her using a gun in here. Too messy.*

Irmgard returned with a book, which she placed in front of me. It was *Final Exit,* the how-to-kill-yourself guide that caused a sensation when first published. Intended purely for an audience of terminally ill patients and their caregivers, it had shocked the general public with its frankness and specificity. Concerns that the suicide rate would rise turned out to be unfounded, but the book's subject matter remains polarizing. I had heard of the book but never seen an actual copy.

Leafing through, I saw many dog ears and highlights. I put it back down, but not before glancing at the copyright date. The thing was almost fifteen years old.

"So, I take it you're going to follow the advice in here in some way?"

"Yes, that's my plan."

"And you're going to do it here? In your condo? And I'll have to find you?"

"No, Tina, that's not what I'm going to do." She paused. "The book suggests doing it in a hotel. I don't want you to have to be the one to come in. And hotels know how to deal with situations like this."

Maybe. But I'll bet they're not giving the housekeepers a lot of hands-on training.

"The authors give advice on methods in here, too," she continued. "You can see I've highlighted sections. I'm supposed to put this book on the nightstand when the time comes, so that there's no doubt it was suicide. The last thing you or I need is this turning into a murder investigation."

"Wouldn't that be ironic?" I muttered, thinking of unforeseen possibilities. "But the advice is old. How do you know it's still accurate? What if their suggestions are outdated? What if somebody tried something and it didn't work? What if there are different laws now?"

"I don't really think it matters, Tina."

"It might. What if what used to be legal isn't anymore? Or what if there are less painful ways? I think you should get the most recent version of this. Really." I paused. "Then you can look through that and tell me as much as I can tolerate hearing about what you decide."

Irmgard ordered the newest edition of the book online that afternoon.

In retrospect, this conversation reverberates with the surreal. How could two seemingly normal individuals, mother and daughter, talk with such rationality about an impending suicide?

In fact, Irmgard and I had long avoided these subjects for that very reason: speaking calmly about such an emotion-laden topic seemed impossible.

But we needed to discuss these details in order for me to participate more fully in the experience of what Irmgard was planning. Either I would stand outside the realm of her decision-making process and feel shut out, or I would have to become involved, diving in over my head and sinking or swimming in the morbid details. There was no wading in for me.

DESPITE THE MENACING STORM on our horizon, my mother and I experienced several exquisite months. They were the kind usually reserved for those with ill or dying loved ones, except we were able to enjoy them in full health.

Knowing each new day represented a chance to be together that we would never have again, we grew closer, something neither of us had thought possible. Moments in time seemed more clearly focused, less blurred by past regrets or future worries.

At some point, I decided that instead of putting flowers by her picture to honor her memory when she died, I would buy her a bouquet every week while she lived, some small part of me still hoping I would be able to continue this new tradition for years.

My largesse embarrassed her, but I know she also savored the attention. She usually had me leave the flowers at the front desk of her building, so her daughter's devotion would not go unnoticed by staff and other residents. And no one could have gotten more pleasure out of those blossoms than she. Not only their colors and shapes impressed her, but also the shadows they made on the wall in the morning sun, and the patterns produced by their fallen leaves. She cherished all of them, even lilies so past their prime that their sensuous white petals curled backward upon themselves, unashamedly revealing their pink, striped secrets. She carefully displayed these in delicate porcelain vases—her "Georgia O'Keeffe flowers."

For years we had talked on the phone, frequently every day. Now we conscientiously called each other every morning and every night. She jotted down lists of occurrences to share with me. These often included the smallest details that brought her moments of unadulterated pleasure: the glistening frost on the fields during her early-morning walk, or the downtown buildings outside her bay window turning to molten gold while reflecting an especially clear sunset. Once she enthusiastically related how a particular ray of morning sunshine had refracted its determined way into her bathroom, although not only a long distance but also three corners separated the nearest window from the shower stall where she was bathing.

My mother observed these miracles every day, the extraordinary minutiae that made the time she had left more superbly, delicately worthwhile.

WITH LUCK, THE RECOLLECTION of all we have encountered during life can keep us company until the end. "Making memories," my mother called the deliberate process of creating lasting remembrances, and throughout her life she studiously set about this task. Enjoying lunch at a restaurant she couldn't afford for dinner or adding candlelight to a meal served at home; drinking tea in a five-star hotel lobby to soak up the atmosphere or window shopping on Madison Avenue; touring Vermont by bicycle, arriving late at every night's destination because she felt no need to rush past the stunning countryside—my mother taught herself to make the most of life.

She also taught herself to enjoy what she had. Her brothers were all financially better off than she. She could have made herself miserable by constantly wishing for more. Instead, she determined to make the best of her situation. She saved for one vacation a year and then lived for the rest of the time off the recollections. Because she didn't cook, she converted her kitchen into a museum of her travels, with beautiful postcards of places she had visited propped up against the wall of the breakfast nook and framed photos of other meaningful locations on the walls.

My mother had not yet fully embraced my need for emotional validation, nor had I yet forgiven her for her planned desertion. Nevertheless, we both vigorously pursued her tradition of memory making in the last months of 2004.

To facilitate our project, I took at least one day a month off from work so we could make day trips to nearby places. During one outing I took one of the most beautiful photographs I have of her, while we waited for our lunch at a restaurant on the Chesapeake Canal. Irmgard is wearing a dark blue blouse with white polka dots. Her hair is parted exactly in the middle and falls delicately below her chin line. Her hands rest on top of each other, supporting her head. Typically, she isn't smiling. Her bright blue eyes are looking to her left out a large plate-glass window onto the canal, watching for a huge cargo ship she is sure will make a dramatic impression on me as it passes. It never appeared, but I treasure the captured moment of her anticipation—and the mood it recalls.

My largest contribution to our memory cache, however, had to do with her seventieth birthday. We both knew to cherish the day, since only my insistence that she postpone her original death date enabled us to experience it. I wanted to outdo myself, to have this be the celebration she, and more particularly I, would never forget. What we didn't know was how sharing such a meaningful occasion would help us recognize that the nature of our relationship had fundamentally changed.

My master plan hatched itself out of Irmgard's love for the architect Frank Gehry's work. For a prior occasion I had bought her a picture book about his buildings, and in it were drawings of the then-unfinished Walt Disney Concert Hall in Los Angeles. The WDCH, as it is known, had since opened, and I wanted to take her there.

I saved enough money for a long-weekend trip for two to L.A. and bought tickets to a baroque concert at the hall. Although I had fantasized about whisking her away to the airport with only "Pack for warm weather" as a clue, I realized that half the enjoyment for her might well lie in planning the trip and picking the sites she wanted to see. So I told her early on, surprising her with a guidebook and telling her about the tickets. She couldn't have been more thrilled at the idea of going to a city she had resigned herself to never seeing.

I booked a room at the once spectacular Bonaventure Hotel. As a young teenager, I had held it in high regard when its four glass towers appeared in movies as a symbol of Los Angeles. By the 2000s, its glory was well behind it, but consequently I was able to afford a two-room suite. Despite the fraying carpet, it felt opulent. After unpacking, we decided to explore our new neighborhood by, of all things in L.A., public transportation. In fact, the entire weekend we got around by bus, which I never would have dreamed possible in a city known for cars. But the plans had been left to Irmgard, who had discovered a means of honoring her lifelong dedication to eschewing driving whenever possible.

In the afternoon light we strolled along streets lined with tall office buildings in order to wander around the WDCH's exterior. There, I too fell in love with Gehry. The building's reflective metal curves drew me into an otherworld of beauty extending beyond time. Irmgard indulged with me, pretending we had the structure to ourselves as we slid through its crevices.

The next day we spent at the Getty Center, L.A.'s famed modern art museum. During the long bus ride, each of us shyly owned up to the fact that we didn't particularly like museums. But by the same token, we both admitted we could never get enough of architecture. Therefore, we decided to remain true to ourselves and ignore the comparatively unappealing inside in favor of the awe-inspiring outside. We drifted the entire day under the smoggy sun—strolling through the gardens; seeking secluded balconies to avoid the crowds; reflecting our images in the ponds, streams, and fountains; and sitting side by side on the cool travertine. Here, I fell in love for the second time on the trip, this time with the Getty's architect, Richard Meier.

That day was Irmgard's birthday, and when we returned to the hotel I treated her to dinner in the revolving restaurant at the top, a view of the city at our feet.

The sun shone more brightly on our final day on the beach at Santa Monica. We not only walked endlessly along the cliffs, the shore, and the pier, but we also rented bicycles. I'll never forget the image of my mother on her bike, helmet perched high on her head, handbag slung around her neck, pedaling hard as she wove through the sand and laughing as she pictured herself. "I look like a monkey on a grindstone," she giggled in German, and I couldn't disagree. But ungainly as she was, few people out there that day were having as good a time as that seventy-year-old simian and the daughter following right behind her.

The final evening, as we changed out of our sandy clothes and into our concert attire, we regretfully acknowledged the conclusion of the celebration. Our glorious respite from reality had been brief, symbolic of our remaining time together. We knew if Irmgard had her way, we would soon have many more endings. The last vacation. The last walk. The last meal. The last touch . . .

While putting on her shoes, my mother admitted, "Tina, you have always been my favorite traveling companion. But somehow this trip has been different. It's not simply that we get along better when we are away from home. But somehow I, who have always been fiercely protective of having my 'space,' am entirely content to share all the space that I have left with you."

This subtle, nuanced change in her attitude toward me confirmed how much our connection had deepened. She was beginning to embrace me, pain and all, and I accepted her, determination and all, as the chosen, worthy companion on the final leg of our shared journey.

We had separate seats for the performance, as I had only been able to find two single tickets. We met at intermission and switched locations. During the second half I sat downstairs in the orchestra section; Irmgard sat in the upper balcony. I never would have believed anyone up there could have heard the final, faint echo of the last violin—except that the woman who told me she heard every note was my mother. And I knew I could believe her now.

IN THE FINAL MONTHS, we shared more than our trip to L.A. For Thanksgiving that year she and I traveled, in a grand, concluding gesture, to Paris. But after Paris, my mother began to wind down her life. She no longer wanted to be gone from home overnight and gradually began to feel the pressure of carrying out her "final exit."

We celebrated Christmas and New Year's together quietly. She purged dramatically, throwing out more letters and documentation. More and more often when I visited her condo, we spent some of the time together going over her plans. She slimmed down her filing cabinet to one half drawer. She made lists of people to contact with the news of her death. She wrote letters in German I could copy and send to her friends. She picked out an urn for her ashes online and had it sent to her.

In those days we treaded lightly around each other so as not to kick up any unnecessary feelings. I kept my tearful moments to myself, and I never, ever saw *her* cry.

I experienced the end of 2004 as exceptionally bittersweet. On the one hand, I felt content in my mother's presence. I appreciated our new understanding of companionship. But that new recognition and acknowledgment could not abate my grief. I longed vainly for something to console me.

But I could not be comforted.

Chapter 13

In an Instant

2005

In July 2005, my father finally moved out of his big house in Wilmington and into the empty condominium I owned nearby. Although the decision had been difficult to make, he felt relieved. His life would have more freedom, and he could begin to enjoy retirement.

But that was not to be.

At work on a Tuesday in mid-September, I received a late-morning e-mail from a woman who lived in my father's building. Reading the note, I immediately suspected something had gone horribly wrong. She had seen Hans sitting outside the building at two on Saturday morning when she returned from a late night out. Afterward, when she left again to walk her dog, Hans had still been in the same position. Upon her return, she found him trying to use his keys to enter someone else's door. "Honestly," she told me later, "I thought he was drunk." She helped him up to his unit and opened the door for him.

Since then, his car had not moved.

I had called him a number of times that weekend. My brother had also called. Hans had not picked up, but that was not out of the ordinary. He led an active life and was frequently not home. I only found it odd that he hadn't responded to the messages on his machine. I chalked it up to his recent bad mood and did not worry. He had acted strangely during the summer, since moving out of his house and into the condo. On Monday, when he still had not called me back, I began to sense something might have happened. *If I don't hear from him tomorrow, I'm going to drive down there after work to check*, I decided.

Immediately after reading the e-mail, I phoned Hans's downstairs neighbor, who by sheer coincidence happened to be a registered nurse.

"I'm really sorry to ask," I explained, "but I just got an e-mail from the woman who lives upstairs. She said she saw my father acting strange very early Saturday morning. She said his car hasn't moved at all since then. I was wondering whether you might have a minute to run upstairs and just knock on his door?"

"I have to go to work shortly, but sure, I can run up and check. Look, I'll do that right now and call you back in five or ten minutes, okay?"

"That'd be great. I really appreciate it. This all just seems a little unusual to me, you know, and I'm a little worried about him since he lives alone."

"No problem. I understand."

I waited forty-five minutes for her call. When the phone on my desk finally rang, I picked it up to hear her crying.

She had gone up to Hans's two-story unit and found his front door ajar. No one answered when she called out as she entered. Not finding him on the first floor, she climbed the stairs to the second. As she turned on the landing, she saw his body. He was lying in the linoleum-floored hallway between the upstairs bathroom and the washing machine.

By that time, he had already been unable to move for approximately eighty hours.

The help Hans had received from his other neighbor in the wee hours of Saturday morning had not been particularly good luck. During the course of that day, Hans's cranium had slowly been filling with blood from a massive hemorrhagic stroke. No one he had interacted with realized this, and he hadn't realized it himself. Had the neighbor not seen Hans or had she ignored his odd behavior, he would likely have fallen down somewhere outside, where he almost certainly would have been found the next morning. Instead, he fell to the floor in his own home and lay there, unseen but not quite unconscious, for the next three and a half days.

Later, when I listened to his answering machine, I found the messages my brother and I had left. We lightheartedly passed the time. We asked how he was doing. We wished him a good weekend. I hope he wasn't able to hear our words as he was lying on the floor. I hope he never even heard the phone ringing. But who knows? As one piece of good fortune in all of that, he did not remember a thing.

I can't forget the first sight of him in the emergency room, where I reached him about two hours after the initial call. He lay on an examining table, cloaked in white sheets and blankets, intravenous lines snaking around his arms. His mouth gaped and his dentures had been removed. He had several days' growth of beard on his chin, caked in places with what I assumed was dried vomit. From his open mouth issued a deep, racking snore. Though he was sound asleep, his wide open eyes stared unseeingly at the ceiling.

When the neighbor who had found him had called me, she held the receiver to Hans's head, and he was able to speak coherently. I told him an ambulance was coming to take him to the hospital and I would be there soon. He responded, pausing between each word, "You . . . don't . . . have . . . to . . . come . . . It's . . . not . . . so . . . serious."

In the hospital, he did not respond to anything. While waiting for the results of the CAT scan, I pulled a chair close to his bed and knelt on it, stroking his face. Unsure whether he could feel or hear anything, I wanted to comfort him on the chance that he could.

Because his stroke had originated in the right frontal lobe, it affected Hans's non-dominant side. He could not move when he fell in the condo because when he collapsed, he fell onto his dominant right side, the only side over which he still had muscle control. His own body weight effectively pinned him to the floor.

I learned later that by the time he arrived in the emergency room, he had lived through the worst of the stroke. If it were going to kill him, it would have already done so. Now kidney failure, or the large and deep pressure sores on his right shoulder, ribs, hip, and thigh presented greater dangers.

But none of these things killed him, either.

Hans spent seven days in the hospital, the first few in intensive care. He might have stayed up to a week longer, but I resolved to get him out as soon as possible and into the Quaker Community, where he had originally wanted to move.

In that type of situation, every patient needs an advocate, and I became Hans's. Pushing against tides of inertia on both the hospital and the retirement community sides, I negotiated assertively on his behalf. Elbowing my way into conversations, paging doctors, and chasing down social workers in the hallway became my standard mode of operation until I finally had in my hands the necessary written permissions to transfer him. When she saw Hans being dressed in preparation for leaving, the nurse on his unit commented to me with surprise, "You are very persistent!"

I chose to take it as a compliment, although she may not have meant it as one.

HANS'S WEEKLONG HOSPITAL STAY began the most difficult months of his life as well as my own. It also marked the start of a very slow and unpredictable journey for us both.

From the moment he was found, it was clear that Hans would not be able to resume a normal existence. The stroke had robbed him of a large part of himself. He could never again be someone's source of protection, stability, or guidance. He was no longer self-sufficient, and although I initially saw my position as temporary, I became his primary and permanent support. My life became tightly and inextricably intertwined with my father's.

Circumstances forced us, unprepared, into new roles. He could be nothing more than a relatively passive partner in any undertaking, and because of this I pushed myself to do the emotional and physical work for both of us. Eventually, I allowed my chosen responsibilities to drain me, until I reached a point where nothing seemed more peaceful than the thought of complete abdication of absolutely everything.

To transfer Hans from the hospital to the retirement community, I drove him myself. Hans sat next to me, and on our trip I quizzed him about the passing landmarks. "What do you think of when you see that?" I asked, pointing.

"Korean grocery. Sushi," he slurred, correctly.

"That's right!" I beamed. "How about that road? Do you recognize it?"

"Route fifty-two."

"Exactly!" I was amazed by what he had retained.

When I entered the long road leading to the Quaker Community's front entrance, I asked again, "Do you know where we are?" Hans said the name of the community and stared at the shrubbery and trees that bordered the building. The deep green of summer was just beginning to fade into dark brown, heralding the arrival of autumn. As I pulled into the circular drive in front of the low, white clapboard entrance, two nurses appeared, waiting to take charge.

HANS STARTED OUT AT the Quaker Community as the model resident. His friends who already lived there came to visit him in the nursing facility section, trying to elicit his interest in books, newspapers, movies, or the bright outdoor courtyard. Other friends drove there every week to sit with him. People brought him plants and his favorite flowers. And Hans, although not consistently charming, earned the staff's respect, for no one in his condition had ever responded so well to treatment.

At first he couldn't speak clearly, and since there was a risk of choking because of the paralysis the stroke had caused, he was not allowed to eat solid foods or "drink" liquids that had not been thickened to pudding consistency. Neither could he walk or sit up by himself. Although he showed little initiative on his own, he worked daily with physical, occupational, and speech therapists. As his recovery progressed, he insisted on using his left side more and more, even though doing so made life more difficult for him. And thanks to careful monitoring and excellent care, the dangerous, stinking, green pressure sores on the right side of his body also eventually healed.

In this process, his training and instincts facilitated his recovery. The stress-reduction business he ran after retiring from Du-Pont involved helping people recover from physical disabilities. Now he worked on himself. To everyone's utter amazement, by the end of October he was climbing and descending stairs unassisted, eating and drinking normally, and performing many grooming tasks. I even have a video of him picking up a yardstick and having a "duel" with the physical therapist. There was talk of his moving into assisted living.

Problematically, this happy prognosis led everyone to ignore that the stroke had exacerbated Hans's character shift. The previously undiagnosed, much smaller stroke earlier in the year had already changed him, and this larger one only made things worse. The first weeks in the nursing facility, Hans appeared subdued because he took anticonvulsant medication and because his brain was still recovering from the enormous damage the influx of blood had wrought. As he regained his physical capabilities and the physician tapered off the medication, his temperament reverted to the anger of the summer. This time the feelings were more extreme and his cognitive deficits even more pronounced.

I learned quickly not to ask Hans where to look for important or relevant documents; he reacted with anger and confusion. I found the title to his car on the floor of the condo, near the trash, in a pile of miscellaneous letters and bills. His will and other papers were shoved into a drawer in his bedroom. The disorganization that followed his first stroke made navigating the intricacies of his former life even more difficult.

I had to accept the fact that this was not going to get better. Hans now had dementia.

What an irony! The fate that my mother went to extreme lengths to avoid. The caretaking she did not want to endure. The suffering she was not able to imagine facing.

All of it thrust instead upon Hans.

HAVING NO SHORT-TERM MEMORY completely impeded Hans's ability to learn anything new. He could understand something in the moment, but within the hour he would forget all about it. Thus, his unrest grew. Over time, he became increasingly vocal and physical in exhibiting his frustrations.

The staff and I learned to try and shield him from potentially disturbing information, but disturbing is a relative term. Letting him watch a spy film, full of intrigue and evil undertones, was an obvious no-no. He perceived enough innocent actions as malevolent without this type of encouragement. But I thought watching an opera performance on TV would be innocuous enough.

As I sat by his side one evening and stroked his hand while we watched *Don Giovanni*, however, I noticed he became increasingly agitated.

I leaned in close to catch his words and heard, "I can't understand a word he's singing. You know, this just proves what I was thinking. It's a conspiracy. I'm being brainwashed, and now I can't even understand English anymore."

Uh-oh, I thought. *The lyrics are Italian.*

"Hans," I interrupted, "I think there are still some cookies over in the lounge. What do you think about going over there to get some?"

"Good idea," he agreed, immediately distracted.

Thank goodness the stroke didn't affect his sweet tooth, I thought as I wheeled him away from the TV. Obviously, I had a lot to learn about how my father now perceived the world.

Generally, Hans found his situation incomprehensible. For one, he thought he still lived in the condo, a private space with locks on the doors. So he could not understand why people constantly roamed the halls, made noise and, worst of all, unconcernedly walked into his room after knocking. He attempted to use the phone but could not grasp that he needed to dial nine first. He wanted to drive but could not find his car. I gave him his wallet with a token twenty dollars inside, but he said he needed more money. His date book gave him no solace, because he could not comprehend the meaning of the entries.

Paranoia ruled his days. He believed staff members colluded to monitor his existence and had "electronically programmed" his bed with "dangerous information." He became irate at any mention of "that damned stroke story," which he suspected people used as a ruse to keep him confined. Such paranoia was consistent with his psychiatric diagnosis of stroke-induced vascular dementia. But the diagnosis didn't lessen his distress or his desperate attempts to make sense of his predicament.

I floundered in these new waters almost as much as he. And, of course, I had a life outside of caring for my father. I had my relationship with Ron. I had a full-time job to hold on to, and a graduate course to teach one evening a week. Also, I had power of attorney for Hans's affairs and had to regulate his legal, financial, and business concerns, all without the help of the person around whom all of this revolved.

I took full advantage of the Family and Medical Leave Act of 1993, which requires U.S. employers to provide up to twelve weeks per year of unpaid leave to employees who take care of family members. I was grateful for the legislation. I took Fridays off, thereby cutting my pay by twenty percent.

Unfortunately, after my father's immediate crisis passed, my continued absence disgruntled my employer. Subtly but persistently, it was made clear to me that time not in the office was considered time poorly spent. Worse, it was expected I would make up the missing hours, resulting in eighty percent pay for one hundred percent effort. But I needed the job, so I tried not to think about it too much.

Despite my struggles, my situation by no means fell at the extreme end of the "sandwich generation" spectrum of possibilities. Ron and I had no children, and Hans did not live with us. When I returned home, no other responsibilities assailed me. Nevertheless, although many younger people act as caregivers to multiple generations, in my immediate circle of friends, I was the only one in this position. My friends talked about marriage, pregnancy, play dates for the little ones, and how to balance home life with an upwardly mobile career path. In contrast, my world now revolved around living wills, nursing homes, dementia, and death.

I was lucky to have Hans living in a place with capable staff. But in those days I felt exhausted, having unnecessarily shouldered too much of the burden. In retrospect, I should have delegated more. I hardly ever asked for help. I made excuses to myself, telling myself only I possessed the legal rights to make certain decisions. But in reality I believed I could do things better for Hans than anyone else. *I am his daughter. I know him best. I know what he needs.* In addition to calling him regularly, I made the forty-five-minute drive to visit him four or five times a week and wrote lengthy updates on the website I had created to keep his friends informed about his condition. I bought Hans clothes, ran errands, and befriended the staff. I ignored my own needs and Ron's, because I wanted to do everything I could in a trying and unforgiving situation.

Additionally, a new behavior almost completely unknown in the pre-stroke Hans disturbed me. Hans now willingly and ably thrust an emotional knife exactly where he knew it would hurt me the most. And he seemed to enjoy doing it. How that shocked me.

"Tina," he said one evening when I called to check in after having just visited, "why are you bothering to call me? You never come to see me. It's obvious you have better things to do than to think about me. Who needs a daughter like you?"

Or frequently when I was with him, he lashed out accusingly, as though I were responsible for his circumstances: "Where is my car? Why are you hiding it from me? You always said you and I were friends, but now I see what you're truly made of."

To his face or on the phone, I maintained control in these situations. But often, rounding the corner of the hallway leading from his nursing home room, I broke into a run for the bathroom. There, in the bright light and stark surroundings, I ran water in the sink so the staff would not hear me crying. Over and over I told myself, "It's not Hans. It's the stroke. He doesn't know what he's saying. He's doing the best he can." Ron held me in his arms at night and repeated the same words: "Brain damage. Dementia. That's not your father talking." But Hans's digs never completely stopped hurting because they were spoken with Hans's voice, with Hans's inflection, and because they reflected an intimate knowledge of my vulnerabilities. This version of Hans knew so perfectly how to punish me that I often felt I was caring for a doppelgänger.

YET HANS ALSO EXHIBITED true compassion for me. During one visit, as I knelt down to tie his shoes, he put his hand on my head and said gently, "Tina, don't overdo it. You're working too hard. You need to take some time out for yourself." How he sensed that I was burning the candle at both ends, I don't know. But he did, and those words brought back the father I had known all my life.

Impaired though he was, Hans sensed what I did not. My working so hard did me no good, and neither did my self-imposed sense of responsibility. My friends listened sympathetically to my troubles. Lucy counseled me every week on the phone. My brother pitched in with visits to Hans. Ron supported me to the best of his ability. I knew people who had cared for loved ones under much more trying circumstances. But I did not share my innermost feelings with anyone and slowly secluded myself in mourning the loss of my cognitively intact father.

Through Irmgard's twenty-year obsession with death, impermanence and loss had become the backdrop to my life. Under the stress of the current circumstances, this mindset warped into a strange variant. I became so completely focused on the seemingly dismal present that I could no longer imagine a future other than what lay directly before me.

Only now do I call my state of mind in those months after Hans's large stroke what it really was: clinical depression. At the time, I simply referred to it as being overwhelmed. The notion of depression seemed out of character with my view of myself. *I am an optimistic and enthusiastic person. I can sometimes be stubborn and opinionated.*

But clinically depressed? That's just not me.

But it *was* me, truly, increasingly, and life-threateningly.

Chapter 14

Darkness

2005

Beginning in November, just two months after Hans's latest stroke, I felt a new numbness take over. I lost my sense of connection with people around me. I became utterly unable to feel joy, and I was completely certain I would never feel happy again. Grief had been normal; this was not. This was dangerous.

Unquestionably, I felt the burden of caring for Hans and running our two lives simultaneously. Nevertheless, I believe in hindsight that I could have avoided plunging into depression. Instead of expressing my feelings, I denied my unresolved pain regarding the loss of Hans as a father and simultaneously pushed myself to the utmost. I had set out the agenda of "doing my best" for Hans, but my best would have been better had it involved taking more responsibility for myself and my emotions. I could have taken so many other paths than the one I took. That one used more energy than I had. While I plodded wearily along, barely able to keep moving and not watching where I was going, my path led me down a hole I emerged from only by luck.

I certainly could have delegated more. I could have reduced my visits to Hans and saved my energy for the marathon rather than use it all up in a sprint. And once in a while I could have built in a "night off," a time when discussion of Hans or my mother was off-limits, when Ron and I could focus on the future instead of the present. I had already achieved my most vital objective: to place Hans in a caring environment. I should have trusted in that and in the abilities of people other than myself. I should have been less arrogant. I should have listened more to my body and my soul.

Yet at the time I felt I had no other options. When friends suggested alternatives, I came up with reasons why they did not make
sense.

AFTER HANS'S NEIGHBOR HAD found him, I called Ron. He raced
from our small house in suburbia to pick me up at my office in
downtown Philadelphia. Together, mostly in preoccupied silence, we
drove south to Wilmington.

I remember the potholes in the asphalt ahead of us when,
snapped out of his own thoughts, Ron pronounced into the whir of
the passing traffic, "Well, you know what they say . . ."

I had no idea what *they* said. What was *he* saying? Had I blocked
out his voice as visions of my father lying in an emergency room
tumbled against each other? "What? What do you mean? What do
they say?" I asked, befuddled.

Cars flew by in the opposite direction. Ron shifted his eyes from
the road momentarily to glance at my tear-streaked face. He took
one hand off the steering wheel, grasping mine and pressing it
against his thigh. "In sickness and in health."

Ron remained by my side, despite the relatively short period we
had known each other. During many of the months from May 2005,
when we had first met, to that September, Ron had been on a cross-
country road trip. Nevertheless, he and I increasingly felt as though
we had known each other for years. Clocked in real time, however,
our experience of living together was extremely brief.

Nevertheless, every visit to Hans, he accompanied me. Every
task, he offered to help. He urged me to take more time for myself,
to let others carry some of the load. Although he had only met Hans
once before the stroke, to my surprise and relief, he treated the impaired version of my father with as much kindness, respect, and humor as he had the healthy version. As I sank deeper into my funk
of inconsolability, Ron represented my primary connection with the
world. But even my bond with him could not pull me from the brink
of despair.

My depression first manifested itself as a different sort of crying. A small incident would seem to flip a switch inside me, and I

would dissolve into tears. I cried everywhere, irrespective of location or companion. It was a desolate, hopeless crying that brought absolutely no relief. I could not be consoled, because I felt less and less attached to everyone around me. But I refused to acknowledge the darkness of the emotions that precipitated these bouts. I knew the feeling was unlike the grief I had faced before. But I didn't want to say this out loud.

After a while, the negative side of every situation obscured any sense of hope with a suffocating fog. The haze became thicker and thicker, until it concealed both my future and my past, leaving me marooned in the unbearable grayness of the moment. In a horrible catch-22, the present was intolerable because it seemed endless, and it seemed endless because it was intolerable.

I resumed therapy with Sarah, but even there I denied my own desperation. Although both Sarah and my friend Lucy urged me to see a psychiatrist, I refused. I rejected any medication stronger than an anti-anxiety pill. I argued I only needed "something to take the edge off."

My primary care physician listened to my rationalizations and suggested antidepressants. I declined. She asked me whether I had a plan or the means to kill myself. I said I did not, but she still only prescribed ten pills of an anti-anxiety medication. She didn't want to take any chances.

For all the fog, I could not see that I was standing at the edge of a gaping abyss. My days felt dominated by seemingly endless self-sacrifice and inexplicable physical exhaustion. The effort it took to live through each day dramatically outweighed any brief moments of pleasure. I became completely self-absorbed, yet I still denied the absoluteness of my despair. I thought about what a relief it would be to end it all.

My own thoughts about death and my mother's suicide plans could not have been more dissimilar. She had calculated far in advance. My ideas had no basis in logic or relation to a distant future I wanted to avoid. They were spontaneous, born of a present so suffocating that I could not imagine enduring it for one day, one hour, one minute longer.

My suicidal ideas began as abstractions, but all too soon they became chillingly concrete. While chopping vegetables for dinner I pictured plunging the kitchen knife through my abdomen. In the bathroom I looked at the deep tub and imagined lying there, my wrists cut, the blood slowly turning the warm, clear water a dark maroon. Driving to teach a class at night, I envisioned turning the steering wheel and swerving my car head-on into oncoming highway traffic. As the weeks progressed, my fantasies edged closer and closer to action. I apparently still had my instinct for self-preservation, however, because I decided to move the sharpest knives out of the kitchen, packing them away in a relatively inaccessible location. And I asked Ron to take the wheel whenever we drove somewhere together.

But depression always has the upper hand. Despite my precautions, one morning when Ron and I were driving to see my father, I had had enough. As Ron sped the car down the highway, I surreptitiously unbuckled my seatbelt. Holding the end in my left hand, I slipped my right arm out from underneath, nudging myself free from its constraint. The fields of a nature preserve raced by. The asphalt of the road's shoulder beckoned to me. Carefully, so that Ron would not notice, I moved my right hand to the door handle. *One quick movement and I can fling myself out onto the pavement*, I thought. At sixty miles an hour, I was fairly certain my death would be instantaneous. And most important, my suffering would be over. Someone else would have to shoulder my duties. Someone else would have to take care of Hans. I would be free from all responsibility. Splat, and it would be finished. For an extended moment, I embraced that intoxicating, freeing idea.

That moment in the car stretches long in my memory. I argued with myself, and after a time my arguments reduced to monosyllables. Yes. No. Yes. No. YES. Never before or since has the line between life and death seemed as thin or depended on so little. Never has death seemed so attainable, so desirable.

I don't remember how my internal battle was decided. I recall making no conscious decision or winning argument. I simply heard myself say quietly, "Ron, pull over." He did, and that decided it.

I DO NOT LET regret dominate my life. Yes, okay, there's the time in fifth grade when I did not tie my wraparound skirt tightly enough, and in the middle of my class presentation . . . And then, not to forget, ignoring the massive infestation of stinkbugs when our house was on the market probably wasn't the best idea. (The real estate agent told me afterward he had been forced to run ahead of the prospective buyers, whacking the insects erratically and flicking their crushed bodies under the rugs.) Yet even on a second run-through, I would not do many things differently in my life.

But I made a very serious mistake by not trying antidepressants that winter. I was wrong to think my suffering could not be helped. Not every antidepressant works for everyone, but most people can find one that is effective.

When you are in a depression, you cannot cure yourself. You cannot pull yourself up by your own bootstraps. You have no bootstraps. You have no boots. Your feet are bare. And life is an endless road covered with burning coals. Every step you take is excruciatingly painful. Every step not taken is just as bad. It's not the time to be making what-if decisions about medications.

I have never gambled with money, but I gambled with my life. I made it through my experience only by luck. Since that time, I have watched a good friend slip into a similar depression. Thanks to my familiarity with the subject, I knew what to do. I spoke up, and I didn't stop pushing for medical intervention. She could not see her situation for what it was, but remarkably she nevertheless listened. She went to a doctor and explained her friends' concerns. She started on medication, and in a few weeks the haze of her previous life seemed like a dream. With the right care and some good luck, recovery can be quick and amazing.

I never want to experience clinical depression again. But if I do, I hope someone will remind me I almost didn't make it the last time.

IN THE DEAD OF winter, just after the holidays of 2005, just after the time when I had wanted to jump out of the car, and just when I thought things couldn't get any worse, they did.

Although no one had told me anything about it, Hans increasingly manifested his anger as physical aggression toward the staff of the nursing facility. My father was a large man, and when he raised his fist in defiance and threatened to punch an employee—most of the time a small woman—he of course frightened her. For over a month the staff discussed among themselves having my father removed from the facility.

Then, two weeks into January, the head social worker and the chief of nursing called me in to see them. I knew we were going to discuss Hans's situation. I had no idea they were going to pull the rug out from under both of us.

"Given your father's repeated physical threats, the staff members no longer feel safe," the social worker informed me. "We've had a team meeting and reached a decision. We're giving you thirty days to find another facility for your father."

He's done what?! I thought. To maintain decorum I said, "This comes as a bit of a surprise. What exactly did he do? And how long have you been considering this?"

"Well, he's threatened some of the staff. They have been complaining for a few months now."

Funny, no one ever said a word about this to me. "I see," I said, suddenly overcome with the urge to leave the room as quickly as possible before I burst into tears. I listened to a few details and then pushed back my chair. I thanked them for giving us a grace period. Only later did I learn that state law mandated the thirty days they offered.

Ron and I spent a soul-searching evening discussing this new development. We both worried about my delicate state of mind and wondered whether I could take the additional pressure this situation would place on me. In order to have the time to find a new facility, I would have to take a vacation from work. I could not delegate this task. Circumstances demanded another stint of concentrated effort, but would this situation end with me throwing my life on the sacrificial altar?

Ironically and indirectly, Hans helped me decide how to balance my needs and his. As Ron and I lay curled in bed that night, I felt Ron's body encircling mine from behind. Protected and feeling at peace for an instant, I closed my eyes and pictured my father's life and mine as it had been on that September weekend when this nightmare began. I pictured Hans lying on the floor of the condo and tried to guess the thoughts that went through his head during those interminable hours. He may have been terrified. He may have been in pain. He may have tried unsuccessfully to get his body to move. But knowing Hans, I couldn't believe he would have contemplated only the negative aspects of his life. Facing probable death, how could he have comforted himself except with thoughts of love?

I then realized that, without a doubt, Hans would never want me to value his life over mine. Visualizing him lying there in the dark, I imagined him addressing me using words he had already spoken. "Tina," he declared, "you have a life to live. You're working hard caring for me. But don't overdo it."

We all have lives to live, none more important than any other. Finally, I understood what he had told me the day I tied his shoes. It had been a message from the depths of his heart.

Hans would be okay. I needed to make sure I would be as well.

Chapter 15

Saying Goodbye

2005, 2008

One moonless evening in early January 2005, Irmgard and I sat together in her living room, holding hands by the light of a small Tiffany lamp. Only a week earlier she had told me the exact date of her planned suicide: Wednesday, February second.

As I turned her hand over in mine, Irmgard took off the ring she was wearing and placed it on my finger. "My fingers are getting thinner," she complained, "and I'm always worried this is going to slip off without my noticing. Why don't I just give it to you now?"

"Are you sure?" I asked, slowly turning the delicate black-and-gold band I had seen so often. I knew the ring well, but it occurred to me that I had only the faintest recollection of how she came by it. "Where did you get this again? Didn't somebody give it to you?"

As Irmgard started to answer, the sudden realization hit me that soon I might lose all her stories forever. Like the time during the war when she and her brothers had slept in beds under a leaky roof in the spare office of her father's factory because they had been kicked out of their house. Wasn't there something in that one about going to bed with open umbrellas to keep off the rain? Or the account of her mother in a movie theater when an air raid started. She ran home through pitch-black, deserted streets, thinking only of her children alone in the house. When she reached the front steps, a bomb fell . . . but what happened next? I suddenly couldn't remember. Or all the descriptions of my childhood. What had been my first word? What had I worn as my first Halloween costume? How had I reacted to the move from Toledo to Wilmington? So many questions left. So little time.

I seized the moment and pulled her from her chair. "Come with me. Where do you keep your jewelry?" I asked. "All of it, even the stuff you don't like so much. Isn't some of it in the desk?"

The next few hours I had her chronicle the history of every piece of her jewelry. We picked up each item and examined it, and I wrote down its story as she told it. Her parents had given her a small diamond ring when she moved to the United States for the first time. When I admired it, she scoffed, "I'm glad you like it. I never did."

"Because you got it from your parents?" I asked.

"No, because they asked me what I wanted and then didn't listen. I wanted something simple and low. I worked in a lab and didn't want something that would catch on things. Instead they got me this, which is tiny and sticks up too high. It was typical: get me something, but not what I want."

Another ring had a different tale. "This one," she said, fondling a smooth black stone set flat in a gold band, "was my first purchase with my own money after we moved to Wilmington. I remember the store where I bought it, a small artist's studio in New Hope, Pennsylvania." She smiled. "It's *exactly* what I wanted."

That evening these random objects, some with intrinsic value, others with none, became holders for our memories. She passed them on to me as gifts, and as I wear them now, they remind me of the history she had with them and of the feelings with which she acquired or received them. But mostly they remind me of that magical evening, as we sat in the circle of light on her white carpet, surrounded by shiny pieces of metal and stone, both of us strangely comforted as the adornments of a lifetime passed in an intimate inventory from her hands to mine.

TODAY IS JANUARY 2, 2008, exactly three years since that memorable night. This morning, like every January second morning thus far, my thoughts turn to my mother and me in 2005, as we moved through the weeks leading up to her chosen date.

As I step outside, the temperature of the crisp New England morning air hovers just above freezing and the scent of last night's receding rain lingers. Dark and ominous clouds cover most of the sky. At the edge of the horizon where the sun has just appeared, the clouds part.

A lot has happened in the past three years. I have switched jobs, moved to Massachusetts, and married Ron. In one way or another, the process I began with my mother influenced many of the decisions I made.

Some of the connections to Irmgard are more casual, however. Take yoga class, for example. I had been attending classes for about a year before the date she planned to end her life. One time I was able to persuade Irmgard to come with me to the YMCA for a session. She took quite seriously the teacher's advice not to push herself when her body told her to stop, and she watched me perform many of the contortions from her default stance on her hands and knees. If she had been an animal, she would have been an ever-tolerant golden retriever, with twinkling eyes and a beaming smile. As I looked over my shoulder or under my arm, I could tell by her indulgent grin that this wasn't for her.

"Tina, I can see why you like it, and I'm glad you like it, but all that stretching is not for me. I'm happy with my walking," she told me afterward.

Yoga is my thing and was never hers, but even now, that memory still ties her to every class I take.

So at seven thirty I sling my yoga bag over my shoulder and set out, happy that I can take this morning walk to class alone, before fellow citizens begin to crowd the streets with their cars and their noise. It is, as my mother often called it, a "Hawaii morning," when the air simultaneously holds the reminder of rain and the promise of sunshine. As I stride quickly along the sidewalk, through my quaint New England town, I think about the former January and February days with my mother.

TWO INTERMINGLED PATHS CAPTURE these moments in my memory. My mother follows one and I the other. The trails intersect frequently at the beginning of the week, when we still saw and spoke to each other. But as twine unravels at the cut end, so my mother and I unavoidably had to unwind from each other. She had her journey to take, and I had mine. And one constant worry echoed in my mind: *For the first time in our lives together, we will not be able to accompany each other.*

Although I still had to function at work and Irmgard insisted on keeping her regular schedule of meetings with friends, and despite being perfectly capable of having phone conversations in which The Day was not mentioned, the coming event occupied an ever-increasing portion of our thoughts. Up to then, we had been able to limit its impact to discussions and consequent actions initiated by my therapy sessions. But as the one-week countdown approached, I felt increasingly out of control.

I'm going to lose my mother, and there's nothing I can do about it. These words attacked me from every angle with escalating frequency. I could only defend myself by having her share with me as much love as possible, as though I could stock up against the coming, everlasting drought.

On the Wednesday before her planned date, I called her from my office just to hear her voice. To my utter surprise, she responded coldly. As if she were standing before my eyes, I could see her backing away from me. She wanted distance, she said, not closeness. This was a difficult time for her (*for her!*), and in order to be able to carry out her plans, she needed to separate from me. She asked me to try to understand.

I panicked. After hanging up hastily, I retreated to the corner of my shared office, and with one shoulder against the closed door, slid down to the floor sobbing. Eventually, my office mate knocked tentatively. I had told her a modified version of the truth, so she was very gentle with me and my volatile moods. After a while I controlled my fears enough to let her in and continue with my day. But I knew my problem with Irmgard had to be solved, and solved quickly. I needed to find a way to have Irmgard recognize *my* overwhelming needs in those last days. Before it was too late.

Back to therapy I went and laid the problem before Sarah. Irmgard and I had an obvious conflict. In order for my mother to be able to achieve her goal, she needed to begin to pull away from the world around her. A person dying slowly does this naturally, gradually losing touch with reality, sinking more deeply into herself, and placidly letting strong attachments and powerful emotions slide by.

My mother had to achieve this through force of will, and I stood in her way.

From my point of view, I faced an entire future without the person I loved more dearly than anyone. I wanted nothing more than to spend every waking moment by her side. My need to create as many memories as possible overwhelmed me. Suddenly, expressions of her love for me seemed few and far between. I craved a constant shower of affection.

These two equally strong desires appeared irreconcilable, and I thought the only alternative was getting Irmgard to see my perspective. After all, hadn't she and I worked hard these past months? Hadn't she begun to respect and understand my position and feelings? The current issue represented simply another opportunity for my mother to step up to the plate.

Sarah had other ideas. To my shock, not only did she understand my mother's position, but she actually supported her right to distance herself from me.

"How do you imagine it feels for her right now?" she asked me. "Can you step outside yourself and try to see these next days from her point of view?"

After some resistance, I tried. "I imagine it's hard. She wants to be with me, and she's still very much alive. I think it's probably difficult to let go of everything all at once."

"And how do you think she feels about you?"

"She probably loves me more than ever," I answered honestly. "And her relationship with me is probably the most difficult thing for her to let go of. But she knows she has to do it if she is going to go through with this."

"And how do you feel about her?"

"I love her more than ever, too."

As we continued to discuss these feelings, Sarah emphasized the differences between the natural process of death and my mother's process. We both came to the conclusion that for Irmgard to successfully separate herself from life, she would need to begin that progression earlier than the final morning. And so we hatched our plan. I had to compromise. My mother would give me the full attention of her love for a few hours, and in return I would give her the distance she needed for her remaining days.

When I presented the proposal to Irmgard, she saw it as a sensible solution to our difficulties. She, too, had been suffering because of our recent friction and was eager to smooth things out. We fixed our date for Saturday.

That day I walked into her condo, prepared simply to tell her how much I would miss her. But my mother had thrown herself completely into this final gesture. She ushered me in, took my hand, and led me into the living room. A flute concerto played on the stereo, and when I stepped into the bright room with the window that looked out onto the city skyline, I saw a pile of pillows arranged on the floor. A few old photo albums lay next to these, as well as a box of tissues. On a small table she had carefully spread a number of silk scarves.

"I thought we could sit on the floor, Tina, and you could put your head in my lap. And I could stroke your hair like I used to when you were little. And I could tell you how much I have loved you for your entire life."

Love. She called it love, not respect, I sighed to myself.

She held my head in her lap and I cried. She told me of her love for me, and through my tears I told her how much I would miss her. She asked, "When will you miss me the most?"

And I replied immediately, "When I'm happy, because I won't be able to share it with you."

She smiled gently at my answer.

For a few hours, I held my mother's complete attention. She willingly listened to all my regrets, heard me describe all the trips I still would have liked to take with her, and comforted me in her arms as I sobbed with grief. I gave her a Valentine's Day card I had written to her. If she stuck to her plan, she wouldn't be there on the actual day, and I didn't want to spend it filled with regret at the missed opportunity. She gave me the scarves she had laid out on the end table.

"Why wait until next week?" she explained. "This way you can wear these and think of me now."

I held her hands for a long time. Caressing them, I felt the softness of her skin and noticed the bony, vein-covered backs, which she always hated and which my father's genes partially corrected in me. I observed the slight bulge of flesh at the end of her fingertips and her subtly shaped nails. I admired one last time her thin wrists, their slightness always emphasized because she moved the buttons of all her blouses closer to the button holes for a tighter, more "shapely" fit.

My mother gave me those concentrated hours as her final gift, and they soothed the ragged tears in my heart more than days interspersed with casual if heartfelt gestures of affection could have. Her caring acknowledgment of my upcoming devastation and of the profound loss she was inflicting on me because of her own desires meant a great deal to me. But that she invited this moment of reflection, focused on my needs rather than her own, at a time when she was in all other ways pulling into herself, affected me most.

She heard me, I thought. She answered with words and small acts that still speak to me now. She opened a space in her heart, let me in, and embraced me with selflessness.

For me, that represented her last true gesture of love.

Following our time together on Saturday came a rapid succession of partings. As though a knife were slowly cutting a hole in my heart, every morning I faced another "last time." The last time we would see each other loomed threateningly on the immediate horizon.

Chapter 16

The Gardens
2005, 2008

Irmgard and I discussed how we would say our physical goodbyes. She let me choose the time and the location. I couldn't bear for it to be in my home or hers. I could not imagine having the ghost of that agony present in my daily surroundings. So I selected one of the distant gardens we visited less frequently, one I had known since childhood. In that place I had many wonderful memories of all the seasons and years that could compete with memories of this event.

This ultimate meeting was important for both of us, but we knew it had to revolve more around me than around her. I would be living for years to come with my memory of these last moments. Her pain would be present only a few more days if she stayed her course.

I took the day off from work. We drove in separate cars and met for lunch in the gardens' café, where we had so often sat before. On that Monday few people occupied the tables looking out over the snow-laden bushes.

What do you eat when you know it will be the last meal you share with someone you love? I ordered nothing more profound than vegetarian chili. Irmgard chose a grilled vegetable sandwich. We talked of foreign affairs, one of her favorite topics, and, for some reason, Meryl Streep. I had brought my camera, and she let me photograph her as often as I wanted.

Irrationally fearful I would forget her face, I intended to take as many pictures of her as I could. Unusually, she acquiesced to my every command: *Look out the window. Warm your hands around your cup. Don't smile; look at me with that serious expression you always wear.* She acted as my totally compliant model.

When we left the building, we turned together toward the secluded meadow path unknown to new visitors. A few inches of snow
covered the ground, but the air was only moderately chilly. Arm
in arm we strode slowly, until we came to the agreed-upon bench.
There Irmgard cleared the snow away from the seat with her mittens
and stomped a firm patch for our feet to rest on. I took more photos,
from near and far. The distancing effect of the camera lens height-
ened the unreality of the moment.

Irmgard was carrying a blue plastic folder. When we sat together,
she produced from it a small, leather-bound diary with gilt edges.
Out of this book, in which she had sporadically written entries addressed to me for over a year, she read from the first pages about her
decision to keep a journal for me, a decision she had made because
she believed I deserved more than simply a final letter. The section
ended with her thoughts about leaving me.

Tina, I'll miss you—a lot! Why? You were always one hundred
percent, totally, on my side.

After the divorce I had steeled myself for the worst, for my
choice had pitted me against everything this culture teaches
us: mothers are hysterical, dumb, old-fashioned, boring, and
dependent. They call too often and get on one's nerves.

None of that from you . . . On the contrary, you always
went out of your way to be with me. And so our blueberry
picking recently was hard for me. So far, I am pretty good
at saying my private goodbyes to places, people, and events.
But, all of a sudden, I realized that I'd like to go blueberry
picking with you again next year.

These are the times when you and I must comfort
ourselves the same way people all over the world comfort
themselves: I will be going blueberry picking with you next
year—in spirit!

After she read her selection, she closed the diary and handed it to
me. Neither of us said anything. We held hands and gazed at each

other's face. I tried to memorize details: her cheeks, red from the cold; her sparkling blue eyes; her lip, slightly scarred from a fall.

"Tina, I think it's time," she said gently after a while. She rose from the bench.

I rose as well, taking off my gloves. I settled the journal on top of them to protect it from the snow. Irmgard opened her arms to embrace me, and I squeezed her tightly, feeling the barrier of our bulky winter clothing between us. Minutes passed before we separated. I stroked her face one last time with my bare hands as she stood without moving.

"I love you very much," I said. Tears formed deep puddles in my eyes. I felt the complete inadequacy of those words to express the depth of my emotion.

"I love *you* very much, Tina. Thank you for being the most wonderful daughter I could have had."

More words would have belied the seriousness of the rupture that was taking place.

Long before this day I had requested that she remain sitting on the bench while I walked away. Irmgard understood; it symbolized the time rapidly approaching. I needed to know she could let me go, could let me move away, let me move on with my life, while she remained static, simply watching my progression, no longer able to accompany me.

I retreated along the path, in the opposite direction from which we had come, still looking at her. She turned around to face me but did not rise again. She only smiled through her tears, raised her hand, and waved. I waved back, unable to smile. I walked slowly backward, keeping her in sight as long as possible. Eventually the path bent. As I rounded the corner I could still glimpse her hand. Then she disappeared. Behind some bushes farther along I sank to the ground sobbing.

For all her reserve, I imagine she may have done the same.

I WOULD NOT HAVE gone to work two days later, Irmgard's chosen day, had there been a better alternative. But I had none, and I needed something to occupy my thoughts, to force me to act the role of someone living a normal life. I had to continue with the process, with the myriad mundane occupations of mind and heart.

This close to Irmgard's potential end, I had only an infinitesimal hope that she would, at the last second, change her mind; that she would tell me about, not a change of heart or a reversal of plans, but simply a stay of execution. "Okay, Tina darling, I just couldn't do it," I imagined her saying. "We'll have one more year."

I called Irmgard that morning after I had gotten ready. For the last months I had been calling her twice a day. Before I left the house for work and in the evening when I came home, we shared our hopes and experiences. But during this last call I knew she expected me to cry, to fall apart, to cling to her desperately and not be able to hold up my end of our bargain.

In the gardens she had let me go, but she did not think I could do the same. That a mother could let a child go had become the central premise in our relationship. But that a daughter could let her mother go so her mother could move peacefully into death? That would not occur gracefully, Irmgard thought. In fact, she had at one point suggested we not speak on the phone at all after the physical parting. I couldn't agree. I promised I would not be needy and told her I wanted contact with her as long as possible. I think she wanted the same, and in the end she acquiesced. And so we spoke: Monday night, Tuesday morning, and Tuesday night. February 2 was Wednesday morning.

The phone call was effortless. Everything in my voice and my entire spirit conveyed the truth of my conviction: I would somehow survive and even thrive again after my loss. I *could* let her go. Everything she heard from me assured her, "Don't worry about me. I'm going to be fine. You do what you need to do." We spoke for quite a while before she relayed to me her absolute surprise about my fortitude.

"Tina," she said, "I have to tell you I am shocked. Why aren't you crying? Why are you so calm?"

"Because I love you, and this is what you want me to do," I responded, not having to think at all about my answer.

"But I thought you wouldn't be able to control yourself. Honestly, I was dreading this phone call. I thought you would be inconsolable."

"I understand why you thought that. I didn't know how I was going to react myself. But right now it's no problem. It's really just that I love you. I want to do anything I can for you." Even as we spoke of it, my inner peace increased.

"I'm overwhelmed. This is not what I expected. I didn't think you would make this so easy for me."

For the first time in my childless life I experienced what I imagine parents experience more often—an absolutely selfless, transformative outpouring of love. No longer did it matter to me whether she gave me what I needed. The tide of love I felt for my mother washed my selfishness away. I found peace in letting her go. Her needs and desires did not simply eclipse my own but actually became my own. In this last moment, my entire being channeled my love into an invincible strength of character. I became a new person, a better person. I finally understood what power comes from releasing the stranglehold of needing—what power comes from giving.

My response resonated from the depth of my soul: *"This is easy.* How could I not want to do the best I possibly could for you today? Ask me to do anything for you and I'll do it."

And I meant it. At that moment letting her go became one of the simplest, least demanding things she could have asked of me. How much more would I have done for her! With no effort and no regret, I let her continue her journey in peace and with my unconditional support.

ON THE MORNING OF February 2, 2005, Irmgard wrote a note on a postcard I had given her long ago, of moonlit cherry blossoms. She left it propped up on her desk, in an envelope addressed to me:

Dear Tina,
This is how the grass and bushes looked this morning in the gardens, only not in moonlight, but backlit by the just risen sun.

I drove there, right after your overpowering phone call.
Tina, now I no longer have any worries. You will make it.
The timer in the kitchen is ticking to let me know when
to leave. Very soon, I will begin my journey.
One more time: I love you very much. All the best. And
thank you, thank you, thank you.
Your Im

At approximately two in the afternoon, Irmgard turned out all the
lights in her condo, rolled a small, black suitcase across her parquet
entry and out into the carpeted hallway, and locked the double doors
to her unit behind her. After taking the elevator down to the lobby,
she passed the mailroom and carried the suitcase out into the garage, where she put it into the trunk before climbing into the driver's seat of her white sedan. Slowly and carefully, she maneuvered
out of her tight parking spot. Her foot on the brake, she removed the
garage door remote control from its hiding place in the ashtray and
clicked the button. Only after the squeaky door had retracted completely did she step on the gas and pull away.

Three years later, I stand on the steps of the yoga building, looking out toward the rising sun, partially hidden by trees and houses
across the street. My cheeks feel warm from the exertion of walking here, and the biting breeze at my back pushes me to continue—
to march far away into the woods, away from things I have planned
for the day. Away from the memories of that painful time with my
mother and instead into wonderful recollections of the periods with
Irmgard that were not overshadowed by the threat of her loss. I have
relived so many comforting experiences in my mind before arriving
here at the door to the studio, and I want nothing more than to hold
on to the bond uniting Irmgard and me right now.

If I enter the building, I know this incredible feeling of con-
nectedness to my mother will evaporate. After class, the air will
be warmer, the street busier, the sun higher, my thoughts not as
sharply focused. Now, not later, is our kind of morning, and I do not
want to let this moment slip away.

Suddenly, I hear Irmgard's voice in my head.

"It will simply be different," she says gently.

And I know she is right. I should go inside. The passage of time does not make things better or worse. It just changes them. My mother's choices led us both to that realization, and I underwent the transformation that has ensued and continues to evolve. My separation from my mother marked the beginning of my learning to let go while continuing to love.

AFTER THE EXTRAORDINARY PHONE conversation with my mother the morning of February 2, I remember very little. How did I get to the train station to go to work that day? I have no idea. In the office, did I just sit at my desk and do nothing? I don't know. Did I eat lunch, dinner, or breakfast? Probably, but I can't recall.

For years I had likened my situation to being tied to train tracks—that familiar scene from silent movies in which the imperiled heroine flails her arms and opens her mouth in a soundless scream at the sight of the rapidly approaching, soot-spewing locomotive. I was that woman. I knew without a doubt the train would proceed relentlessly and run me over no matter what I did. In my mind, I often saw its black grate almost touching my chest, its massive bulk demanding that all my attention be focused on only the inevitable instant of impact. But try as I might, I could not bear to imagine how life would be after it had hit me, how the collision would not kill but change me. I knew reasonably well the person I was at this moment. But who would I become? And how would that new person go about living my life?

Chapter 17

The Suitcase

2005

In my last words to my mother that February morning, I demon-
strated great selflessness both to her and to myself. In front
of her, putting my own needs aside had been the simplest of acts.
Nevertheless, after I hung up the phone, the finality of the situation sank in. Although I would move with her in spirit through the
day and into the night, if things went as planned I would never, ever
speak with her again. In the face of that knowledge, performing the
simplest tasks of daily life felt incredibly difficult and completely
irrelevant.

Irmgard and I had discussed the irony that the day she was going
to die, she would still put on clean underwear, brush her teeth, and
take out the garbage. Superficially, nothing would be different. For
me as well, her final day would consist of struggling through a mo-
rass of the mundane.

I had deliberately not changed my appointment for a haircut. After that I had an evening yoga class. A trip to a salon and then trying
to relax seemed a little obscene given the circumstances, but anything was better than coming home to my empty condo. Hans offered to let me spend the night in the guest room of his house, but
because of the bitter divorce and their long estrangement, his house
seemed too much like enemy territory for my mother on a night in
which she filled my head and heart. Although I knew my father's
presence could comfort me, on this night of all nights I couldn't
bear to "defect."

That evening the stylist tilted back my chair and began to wet my hair. I stared up at the while ceiling tiles and she asked me, as usual, "So, is anything new going on?" Her question instantly transported me to the random hotel room in the undisclosed location that my mother had chosen for her suicide. Was Irmgard "asleep" by now? I speculated. Would she panic as consciousness began to slip from her grasp? Would everything go smoothly? Would she have regrets?

"No, there's nothing new," I replied. "Days just go by, don't they? No matter what is happening, it always turns into tomorrow eventually." I had intended this to be a lighthearted answer, and it felt comparatively bright to me, given the circumstances. Not to the stylist, however. My answer effectively stopped our conversation. The wash and cut took place in silence, an eerie counterpoint to the chatter all around me and the pounding thoughts within my head.

Freshly coiffed but feeling considerably depleted, I drove to the yoga class. By that time in the evening, half of my brain was screaming, wanting me to confide to the volunteer checking people in at the YMCA, to the yoga instructor, to my classmates, to anyone, the living nightmare in which I was trapped. *Can't they tell just by looking that something is desperately wrong with me tonight?* But no one asked me how I was doing. None of my classmates flashed a concerned glance my way as we contorted ourselves on the mats.

"Remember to breathe," the teacher advised as we held the yoga poses. But even breathing seemed painful, and halfway through the class I had to excuse myself and leave the room.

The gray cement-block wall of the hallway was cool as I rested my forehead against it, finally unable to stifle the sobs that rose in my chest. Turning around, pressing my back against the wall, I slid to the floor and drew my knees into my ribs.

My mother is dying tonight.

The sentence pounded in my head like a drum. My early-morning resolve and courage had vaporized.

There are moments when we wish chronology were not synonymous with change, when moving forward in time did not require us to face unknowns, to become a different person, to watch the present slip inexorably into the past. In that moment on the floor, I knew my mother was still alive. *If only I could keep her alive, preserve this moment in amber, for all my selfish reasons*, I thought. *I don't even have to see her again. Just knowing she is alive would be enough. I don't want to move on with my life alone.*

Irmgard told me she had read somewhere that we do not truly become an adult until our parents die. This rang true with her own experience, and she passed the thought on to me as a solace. Losing her was the first step I would take toward being able to live my life completely as I chose, she said, without the psychological and emotional restraints of being a daughter. What she failed to acknowledge was that I would also lose my primary source of support.

Certainly, I did not think I could ever leave her entirely behind me. I cherished the traces of Irmgard that had taken up residence in my psyche since childhood. But despite the knowledge that part of her would live on inside me, that night the idea of taking the first step onto the uncharted, motherless pathway of my life terrified me.

ALTHOUGH I DID NOT have a stadium full of allies during that time, I did have a few supporters standing on the sidelines. And on the morning of February 3, with my mother in a hotel somewhere in Delaware, I went to work in Philadelphia with two of my colleagues fully aware of what the day had in store for me. I had confided the truth to each of them, and for the entirety of my six hours at my department that day, one of them remained by my side. I had not asked for this physical manifestation of support, but because they felt utterly helpless to give me any words of comfort, they instinctively drew close to me. Strangely enough, I did not realize I had not been left alone—even in the bathroom—until many days later. I only knew I was suffering slightly less than I had thought I would.

That day, every time the phone on my desk rang, I almost jumped out of my chair. *Is this a call from the hotel? Or a call from the hospital emergency room? Or is it . . . could it be . . . Irmgard?* My heart thudded in my ears and my hands became instantly cold, as though my blood had suddenly turned to stone and my heart was trying desperately to circulate it again. Invariably, it was the secretary or

a colleague who had called. My heart raced many minutes before recovering, and even more time passed before the color returned to
my face.

At two thirty, there was an unexpected knock on my office door.

Shaken, I opened it to see my boss, looking very serious. Usually
ready with a joke or a smile, he nodded once and said, "Tina, please
come to my office."

Before I could reply, he had turned around and was walking
down the hallway. With trepidation, I followed. *This is not a good
time*, I wanted to say. *I can't leave my phone unattended. And if this
is about my mother* . . . As I followed him, I worried that if he was
going to tell me my mother was dead, I might not react "appropri-
ately." *Am I going to be able to look surprised?*

I could not manage to say anything and instead plunged my icy
hands into my pockets.

Once he closed his door, he sat behind his large, imitation-
mahogany desk and asked me to take a chair in front of it. With a
grave face, he adjusted his glasses and looked down at his pens. I did
too. As he spoke, each word pierced me.

"I just got a call from the police," he said. "They told me that
they found your mother in a hotel room . . ."

His eyes left the desk and darted around the room, unsure of
where to rest but wanting to avoid mine at all costs. After breathing in deeply, he focused on his folded hands and exhaled the words,
"She's dead."

I needn't have been concerned about my reaction. I had spent
the past thirty-six hours barely daring to inhale, waiting with increasing, excruciating tension for the train I had so long envisioned
to stop or finally run me over. With relief more than anything else I
broke into tears as he shared the content of the brief call.

"Your mother was in a hotel that was paid in advance for the
night. But she never checked out. The front desk called her room a
number of times. There was no answer. Eventually, a manager went
up to the room and let himself in. Beside the body, he saw some kind
of a note and called the police. The police were there a couple of

hours, and apparently your mother's been moved somewhere else." The word "morgue" hung in the air, unspoken.

"Anyway," he continued, "the police thought it was best you hear all of this from someone you know. So they called the front desk, and the call was transferred to me. I think your mother must have left this number. I'm really sorry, Tina." He handed me a box of tissues across the desk.

My first condolence.

Finally, I realized, *I am going to be able to grieve in public.*

IN THAT INSTANT, YEARS, months, and days of inaction and immobility converted into rapid activity. One of my colleagues drove me to my father's house. From the car, I called Hans, my brother, and Lucy. I waited until I was with Hans to call the police.

"How are you doing?" the crisis intervention officer asked. "This must be a big shock for you."

"Well, I'm okay," I said. "But to tell the truth, it isn't a shock. I had the feeling she was going to do this," I continued, fudging the extent of my foreknowledge.

"Oh." There was a pause. "I'm very sorry to hear that."

My second condolence.

"Thanks," I replied.

She gave me the number of the police station that had possession of my mother's effects. When I phoned, the detective in charge of my mother's case asked me to come to the station and answer some questions. I also had to pick up Irmgard's belongings. In addition, he reminded me my mother's car was still in the hotel parking lot.

Hans offered to come with me. Before we left, he and I sat on the sofa in his living room, feeling the need for quiet reflection before the inevitable madness of the next hours. We looked out into the garden where I had played as a child. On the windowsill stood one of my father's marvelous amaryllis plants, in full bloom with four pink-and-white-striped blossoms, reminding me of my mother's Georgia O'Keeffe flowers.

"How are you holding up?" Hans asked, turning to me with concern and sandwiching my smaller hands between his much larger ones.

"I'm better than I thought I would be," I answered. "And I'm very glad I am finally going to be able to do something instead of just waiting for all of this to happen. The waiting was worse than you can ever imagine."

"Well, it was harder for you, because you believed she would do it. I didn't ever really want to believe that she could go through with it."

"I know you didn't," I said, looking out the window again. "What I can't believe is that I'll never see her again."

AFTER A WHILE, WE got up and went to his car. By pure coincidence, the drive to the police station took us directly past the hotel where my mother had died. It was nauseatingly eerie to see the building she had entered alive, just over twenty-four hours earlier. But Hans was a practical German. He suggested we stop there on the way home so I could drive her car back. Reluctantly, I agreed.

We arrived at the station after five. The building seemed deserted, except for the officer manning the telephone at the front desk. Through an intercom I asked to see the person I spoke with earlier. Eventually, a serious-looking man in his early thirties came into view from down the hallway. Tall and clean-cut, with straight, dark hair parted to the side, in his civilian clothing he looked as though he might have been on his way home.

He ushered us in through locked doors. Showing Hans and me into a stark room with two black plastic chairs and a bare wooden table, he gave me his card, which identified him as "Detective Borlag, Criminal Investigations." An impressive title. It panicked me. *Murder investigation, here we come*, I thought. The detective grabbed another chair for Hans and then disappeared.

My mother and I had discussed many times the possibility of the police thinking I had somehow been involved in her death. We wanted to minimize any chance of my becoming embroiled in a murder inquiry, although the idea of my being a suspect was ludicrous to both of us. I was without a doubt the last person on earth who wanted my mother to die, but we realized it might not look that way to an outsider. Therefore, she had taken the precaution of never telling me the name or location of the hotel. I also had no idea of how she planned to take her life; in the end I had asked her to tell me what she was *not* going to do. I knew she would not use a gun, rope, knife, or electrical appliance. We discussed almost everything else, but the specific details we avoided to spare me too real an image. It also meant I was able to answer the detective's questions without deception.

In addition, Irmgard and I had talked about the things she would leave in the hotel room beside her body. On the night table next to the bed, she would leave a note asking the police to call me and giving my office phone number. There she would also set her copy of *Final Exit*, with relevant passages underlined and her name inscribed on the inside.

I had suggested two additions: that she place her driver's license by the bed, for ease of identification, and that she leave a note in the entry hall addressed to the first person to enter the room, warning this person of what she or he would find by advancing farther and advising that the police be called. I did not know whether my last suggestion could spare a housekeeper or the hotel manager any unnecessary upset, but I thought it best to try.

After a long absence, Detective Borlag returned to the small room where Hans and I waited. He lugged a plain brown paper bag with handles and had a bulging manila folder tucked under one arm.

He put the bag on the floor, sat down across the table from Hans and me, and opened the folder. I tried to see what was written on the papers in it, but the table was too wide, perhaps by design.

"As I told you on the phone," he began, "your mother was found dead at the hotel when the management investigated. After they found her, they called us. An officer and I arrived at the scene and found your mother lying on top of one of the beds." He paused and looked up at me. "From your reaction on the phone, I take it that you were not surprised when my colleague told you that your mother killed herself?" he asked.

"No, I wasn't," I answered succinctly.

In front of a police detective investigating my mother's death, I felt intimidated. I could hardly answer his question and was shaking on the inside from nervousness. I held my hands loosely on my thighs, pretending to be calm. Although I believed I had nothing to hide, I nevertheless felt like someone driving at the speed limit who has just been pulled over by a police car with flashing lights and blaring siren. Intellectually I knew I had done nothing wrong, but the circumstances provoked guilt.

Detective Borlag continued. "As I said, we found her lying on the bed. There was a plastic bag over her head and there was a half-empty bottle of vodka in the room. We suspect that she also may have taken some medication, but we couldn't find . . ."

I could no longer listen and hastily interrupted. "I'm sorry. I realize you may have to tell me some of this, and I understand that. But I would really appreciate it if you would keep as many of the details to yourself as you can."

When my mother and I had agreed months ago that I should not know the particulars of her plan, I had been thinking of more than just my own legal protection. I very much wanted to remember my mother as a living person, not a corpse. I did not need to see her dead body or hear how she had killed herself in order to accept that she was gone. Knowing she suffocated herself can still make me shudder today.

Most people have perhaps at least considered what would be their worst-case dying scenario. For me this would involve either drowning or suffocation, and it still turns my stomach that my mother's death certificate states the cause of her demise as "Suicide. Found in hotel room with a plastic bag over the head." It is especially horrifying because this certificate does not stay private: everyone wants a copy, from banks to employers to the Social Security Administration. I faxed and mailed it all over the country.

Obviously, my mother did not feel the same way I did about "asphyxia," as the certificate also declares. Personally, I take comfort in the likelihood that the mixture of alcohol and drugs killed her before the bag did. But *she* had mainly worried about having "an accident," by which she meant *failing* to kill herself. She wanted to avoid causing her body or mind some manner of irreparable, but not fatal, damage. In fact, *her* worst-case scenario was for the hotel staff to find her in a near-death state and call an ambulance, then for doctors to take heroic measures to "save" her, only to doom her to the vegetative state she had gone to such lengths to avoid.

Detective Borlag nodded his head once to indicate that he understood my position on details and then continued. "Do you have any idea why she may have done this?"

I could answer this question more easily. It was my standard mantra regarding my mother's decision. "She planned this twenty years ago. My mother wanted to live a healthy life and then die while she was still healthy. She didn't want to die spending lots of money to prolong her life. She valued quality over quantity. She called it being terminally healthy."

"Was she depressed?" he asked.

"No. Not at all. Just the opposite," I tried to explain. "She was so aware of every beautiful thing around her because she knew she wasn't going to be alive indefinitely. I know maybe it sounds strange, but that's just the way she was. She was very stubborn and wanted to have control of this last thing. It gave her peace."

I don't for a moment think he understood my explanation, but he wrote something down and continued. "Well, I don't know if you know, but suicide is not illegal in Delaware."

"It isn't?" I interjected in disbelief. My mother and I had somehow overlooked this crucial detail.

"No, it is not. And we're treating your mother's case as a suicide. But we need to ask you some more questions. And there may need to be an autopsy on her body, which would mean that it will take longer to get a death certificate."

"I understand." The possibility of an autopsy did not surprise me, but visualizing someone beginning to carve my mother apart,

I hastily repeated to myself that the body in their possession no longer housed the person I loved. *It's just a body. It's just a body. It's not her.* I tried to put thoughts of the medical examiner out of my mind.

As for my reaction to the rest of his statement, I melted with relief. *I am not a suspect in a murder investigation.* Suddenly the room felt larger. My shaking ceased. For the first time since I had entered, I felt as though I had space to breathe.

Our conversation continued for a while longer. My father sat silent, and the detective ignored him. To signal the end of the interview, he gave me some forms to sign. I don't remember what they were, but I do remember my last question.

Summoning courage, for I greatly feared the answer, I asked, "When you saw her, did she look like she had suffered?"

Detective Borlag looked directly at me and replied, "No. Actually, she looked very peaceful."

"Thank you," I said softly.

Hans and I rose and the detective handed me the bag of my mother's things, which he had kindly not gone through with us. He asked us to wait while he retrieved the suitcase my mother had taken with her to the hotel. After he carried it out from a back hallway, I knelt and placed the bag of belongings inside.

Out in the dark parking lot, the stress of the past hour suddenly overcame Hans and me.

On the short path to the car, we started arguing heatedly about, of all things, my mother's suitcase. I wanted to find the nearest dumpster and get rid of it and all its contents immediately. My father, ever the frugal German, could not part easily with potentially useful items. He objected.

"It's a perfectly good suitcase. I'll keep it," Hans exclaimed upon hearing what I wanted to do.

"No," I immediately raised my voice. "You can't keep it. It was Irmgard's. You can't have it. But I don't want to see it. I have to throw it away." It seemed I had left all rationality behind in the interrogation room. I began looking around.

"We have to find a dumpster!" I cried. Then, seeing a trash can near the station door, I ran over to it with the suitcase. The opening was far too narrow to accommodate a maximum carry-on size. "Help me lift off the lid," I yelled to Hans with a frenzied tinge to my voice. "I'm going to throw it in here."

"You can't do that," Hans said, walking over. His voice was also rising in volume. "I said I'll take it. It's a good suitcase." He made a grab for the handle, as I gave up on lifting the lid and tried to stuff the rectangular object into the absurdly small round hole.

I yanked the suitcase out of his reach. "You don't need a suitcase, and I don't want to see what's inside. I don't want to know any more about how she did it!" Tears began to roll down my face. I felt desperate and furious that he could not understand my point of view.

Seeing me cry, my father suddenly calmed. "Look, Tina. How about if I take the suitcase home? I'll unpack it. I'll take the things out. You won't have to look at them. And I'll give the empty suitcase back to you when you want it. You can throw it away then, or you can keep it. It will be up to you. Just don't do it now. Let me take care of going through it."

He reached over and placed his hand over mine. I let go of the handle and he gently took the suitcase from me.

Hans had understood what I had not. My issue wasn't with the suitcase; it was with the items inside that had killed my mother—the vodka, the baggies, and whatever else. I didn't want to touch these things, but I had no personal vendetta against the bag that had carried them.

To signal the end to the argument, Hans opened his arms and embraced me while I wept.

Then he put the suitcase in the back of his car and we drove to the hotel. We snaked around the parking lot for a while, until I recognized Irmgard's white sedan in a corner. She had backed the car into the space carefully, precisely between the white lines. The door was open, and her set of keys was in the glove compartment, just as she had said they would be. I got in and, as always, had to adjust the seat to fit my longer legs under the steering wheel. Once out of the parking lot, I followed the taillights of my father's car along the road.

The interior of the car still smelled faintly of my mother.

I stared straight ahead and took a deep breath. I imagined Irmgard sitting in the seat next to me. Her soft and companionable silence led me toward a place beyond words, beyond reasons, as we drove together into the gathering darkness.

Who am I now that you are gone?

Chapter 18

In Sickness and in Health

2005

No one could have predicted in the spring of 2005 that Ron and I would meet in early summer. If someone had asked Ron's friends about the likelihood of his settling down again, none of them would have thought it probable. True, some harbored secret wishes, along the lines of, "If only he could meet the right person . . ." But since his previous marriage thirty years earlier, Ron had been steadfastly nomadic and only fleetingly attached. His friends had long ago given up real hope.

Based on my experiences with my first husband, I'm not so sure what my friends would have said about me, either.

I willfully ignored the warning signs in my marriage with Sam, remaining together with him for over two years. The emotional reverberations reached deep into my soul. The cycle of our abuse and codependence had been insidious. After we divorced, I developed a sense of pride for having found the strength to end it. In time, I also forgave myself for my role in the problems. But most of all, I sighed repeatedly with relief. I had rid myself of a psychological albatross before the full weight of Irmgard's impending final act began to smother me.

Living alone was a comparative pleasure to the married life I had known. Nevertheless, in the fall of 2004, I came to a realization: I wanted to go out on a date again. I did not necessarily want to find another life partner, although I was open to the possibility. First and foremost, I simply wanted to expunge the memory of my last date with my ex-husband. The idea of going to my grave with Sam's sad face as the last one I had seen over an empty restaurant dinner plate disheartened me.

Unfortunately, I had too little recent experience and too much anxiety. When I finally met the overworked lawyer I had corresponded with online, it represented my First Date in Years. Walking to the restaurant where we agreed to meet, I sweated, my heart raced, and I almost threw up. But it didn't take long to see the gulf between our outlooks, exemplified by his falling asleep during the play we saw after dinner. I pretended not to notice, but I was mortified—not as much by his snoring as by my own anticipatory fears about such a perfunctory undertaking as a date. As he noisily dozed, I silently hoped his nap would not give him a second wind. I wanted the evening over with as quickly as possible. Luckily, his snooze only deepened his fatigue. And by the time he walked me to my car, we both knew we lacked any sort of chemistry.

With the first date behind me, I approached my second and third online adventures with more calm. And when no sparks flew there either, I cheerfully put my dating ideas back into the closet and forgot all about them. I had gained what I sought—new memories on top of the last ones, and a bit more equilibrium.

Meeting Ron resulted from an unpredictable and lucky confluence of events. Although we had grown up in the same area, gone to the same high school, and participated in the same college study-abroad program, we had never encountered each other. Ron was twenty-two years my senior. And our shared indifference about reunions prevented us from meeting in the only other way it would have been possible—before the Internet, that is.

Coincidentally, at the time my six-month membership in the online dating service was expiring, Ron was joining the same service. It was May, and he hoped to use this cyberspace medium to find a companion for a cross-country road trip he planned for the summer. He spent much of his life either traveling around the United States or developing hiking trails, or both, and as part of his newest project, he was searching out a course for a transcontinental footpath that would connect many pre-existing trails across the northern tier of the Lower 48.

Remarkably, he had successfully used ads to find willing female travel partners for even longer trips, so he gave it another try. To him, joining a dating service seemed eminently practical. He probably never considered that the women members might want something more out of a date than the prelude to sharing a hot, dirty van for months on end. But Ron planned a trip to the Philadelphia area to visit his mother, and searching for a partner while he was back home seemed logical: *I'll go visit Mom. While I'm there, I can find a woman who has the next three months free to drive across the country with me.*

Well, okay—maybe that sounds logical only to Ron.

One evening an e-mail from a stranger arrived in my virtual inbox. The message carried an attachment. Fearful of malevolent viruses, I hesitated to open it. *No sense risking my hard drive for the sake of an e-mail.* I checked the delete box and moved on down the list of new mail.

When we think about it today, that act gives both Ron and me shivers. If I had gone ahead with my initial inclination and deleted his e-mail, he would have taken my silence as lack of interest and we would probably never have met.

But because his name sounded vaguely familiar, I unchecked the delete box before shutting the machine down for the evening. *It's the attachment I'm not supposed to open, after all, not the e-mail. It's probably spam, but there's no harm in checking.*

His message was short, choppy, and full of the backpacker jargon that still befuddles and amuses me. At first I had no idea what this fellow was asking. He had found me through the dating service. He apparently lived in La Jolla—or, equally plausible from what he had written, Seattle—and was looking for a "fun companion" for a long summer drive.

The potentially harmful attachment turned out to be a photo of himself. In it he looked like a tall, skinny, middle-aged gnome. Clad in a red raincoat, a floppy, unattractive pink hat, and *very* skimpy bright-yellow running shorts, he was squatting beneath a trail warning sign in a desiccated landscape of orange and gray brush.

Well, I thought, one thing you can be sure of: he's not concerned about making a sophisticated first impression.

Still, something about his smile radiated good humor and ingenuousness. Out amid the scrub, seemingly in the middle of nowhere, dressed in weird color combinations, this man was obviously having the time of his life.

So I took the next step of all savvy Internet daters and Googled him. *Hmm . . . author. Conservationist. Winner of big awards.* I clicked through his website and corroborated some of his claims through online searches. He seemed to be harmless, if obsessively woodsy.

I e-mailed back a polite but clear "no thanks" to his offer of a cross-country trip. Yet something made me add at the end of my refusal, "If you're interested in a less demanding meeting of some type, let me know."

He was. And he did.

Our e-mail correspondence rapidly escalated in intensity. As the first days of our electronic courtship unfolded, I became more and more certain I wanted to meet this man. He intrigued me, and conversely I, apparently, intrigued him. He sent me in-progress chapters of his books. I sent him short essays I was submitting for publication. E-mails began to flow back and forth several times a day. And then he finally flew out to visit his mother and called me during a break in the yard labor she immediately set upon him.

"When my mother sees me, she automatically thinks, 'My boy's back, and the yard needs work!'" Ron informed me during our first phone call. "I'm out here in her garden, helping her plant roses. She's gone inside to get out of the sun, and I thought I would take a moment and call you."

I stood in my office, under a brown-leafed, dying spider plant hanging in my window. To steer the conversation away from horticulture, I asked, "Where does your mother live, exactly?"

"Near Newark, Delaware."

Phew. That meant he was only an hour from my home. "That's a nice area," I said, feigning interest. I had actually never been to any of the neighborhoods around Delaware's one university town.

"My mother's place is okay, but the area as a whole is nothing special. Being near the university is good. I sometimes go there to use the library. Actually, I used to go there all the time to use the Internet until I finally persuaded my mother to get a connection in the house." *Perhaps he was babbling?* "Anyway, I just thought I would call to hear what you sounded like. I probably should get back to the planting."

"Well, I don't want to keep you, but . . ." *Go ahead and ask.* "And I don't know whether you're interested, but since you're not that far away, maybe we could set up a meeting in person sometime?" *Not very elegant, but please say yes.*

"Good idea. I'd like that. Any suggestions?"

Phew, again. I took out my date book and paged through the next week. "Well, having said that, it turns out I'm kind of busy. How about next Thursday night? We could meet somewhere halfway."

"Thursday? You mean a week from tomorrow? That sounds okay."

But after many telephone conversations on subsequent days, I decided I simply could not wait. The excitement building in the relationship was beginning to wake me up early in the morning and keep me up late at night. Although embarrassed by my eagerness, on Saturday I took the plunge and called Ron to suggest an earlier rendezvous.

My call found him in the garden again.

"Tonight?" I could tell he was genuinely taken aback.

"I know it's crazy, but I just thought it might be fun to see each other now. Then, when the time of the real first date comes on Thursday, we can feel more relaxed about it."

He laughed. "You're right. I usually hate blind dates, but I find myself wanting to rush into this one. I can see you after dinner. How's seven?"

We chose the high school we had both attended as the site of our first meeting. We walked around its familiar grounds and the neighboring park, talking for hours about school and friends, past events and present occupations. And foreshadowing the slightly warped "nostalgic" streak I would come to know well, Ron pointed out all the bushes where he and his classmates used to vomit when made to run three miles after lunch for cross-country practice.

As dusk became dark on that initial encounter, we threaded our way through the lamp-lit streets toward the state art museum. Although the entrance was black, we could see light shining from the rear. Someone had rented the main exhibit floor for an event. Sneaking close to the building, we observed the scene through the floor-to-ceiling windows. Women in evening gowns and men in tuxedos silently edged their way toward a buffet. Others sat talking at tables festooned with votives and flowers. Couples swayed romantically to inaudible music, bodies entwined.

Outside, we heard only the cicadas, screeching their own rhythm, completely oblivious to the festivities.

"If you could pick for yourself any gown you can see in there, which one would it be?" Ron asked from behind me, as I became absorbed by the scene.

"Actually," I confessed, displeased at having to admit this so early on, "I don't usually wear dresses. I don't really like them much. But," I countered quickly, "what suit would you pick?"

"I like different ones, from tails to tuxes. But it doesn't matter that you don't normally wear dresses. Which one do you like?"

I scanned the women. Frills and floor-length to sleek and short. But the one I liked the best was simple—a long, flowing gown of red, strapless and elegant.

"That one. The woman standing by the buffet. She's just picking something up."

"Nice choice," Ron said, placing his hands on my shoulders.

My heart beat faster. "Which suit would you pick? You didn't answer."

"That one. The double-breasted tuxedo walking up to the buffet table," Ron whispered as he pulled against my shoulders and pushed his chest into my back. I could feel the buttons of his shirt press into my spine and I leaned, ever so slightly, backward. "Hey," he slid his cheek against my hair. "Did you see that?"

My dress and his tuxedo had just kissed.

That evening Ron and I did not, however. At the end of the long walk, we parted with a friendly hug. But I was hooked, and so was he.

A few dates, many talks, and much laughter later, I spent a lunch hour at work looking up medical journal articles on the chemistry of being in love. But despite my left brain's efforts at pursuing a logical path, science did not play a large role in the interactions between Ron and me. Things proceeded in a more primal, instinctual direction. Despite our age difference and our incredibly discordant life experiences, Ron and I very quickly recognized in each other the person who could bring out the best in us.

THAT'S NOT TO SAY life has been perfect between us since then. We came together and moved in with each other as middle-aged adults, both with firmly established patterns of living and interacting with others. Our love had conditions. And unfortunately the affection we felt for each other initially was stretched beyond the bounds of most early relationships. Loss surrounded me—first my mother's death, then my father's stroke—and I found it difficult to hold on to Ron with any gracefulness. In the beginning I clung, needled, cajoled, and accused, for no rational reason. Sometimes I felt overwhelmed by the baggage of past relationships, most especially my previous marriage. These shaped my expectations, fears, and hidden agendas. Sam may have "set the bar low," as Ron liked to put it, but that didn't mean the relationship with Ron had no invisible hurdles. In the beginning, we'd hit one of them full speed and fall flat.

"How could you do that?" I would assail him.

"What? What did I do?"

"You don't even know? I don't believe it. How can you live with me and still not know? How can you do that and then tell me you don't even know what you did?"

That was when we hit a Tina-constructed obstacle in the relationship.

When we hit one of Ron's design, the indicators were usually nonverbal. He'd simply disappear. I would find him sitting in his van in the driveway, talking to his Seattle friends on his cell phone. Or, claiming work trumped all needs, he would cloister himself in his study.

In retrospect, I am amazed we survived as a couple.

Of course, since Irmgard died in February and I met Ron in May, he had no part in my experiences leading up to and immediately following my mother's suicide. Naturally, all Ron knew of her came from me, and through me he received mixed messages. My words told him I loved her. My actions told him I still suffered because of her selfish decision. After a particularly touching movie, or a disturbing visit to my father in the nursing home, I would clench my arms around his chest and bury my head into the crook of his neck, sobbing for Irmgard. Not surprisingly, Ron came to resent her for having left me prematurely, for knowingly causing me such inordinate pain.

With regard to my father, Ron and I developed a different understanding. Ron's father had died ten years earlier, and Ron had unresolved feelings about him. But in general, he accepted my ongoing and changing relationship with Hans for what it was. Ron realized that because of Hans's problems, I hung on Ron more than I would have otherwise done. Yet we both also strove for something more between us than just mutual need.

With my ex-husband, a million red flags told me to run. Yet I ignored every sign, just as he had ignored the opossum in the kitchen, hoping everything disturbing would just go away on its own. In the end, I had used Sam for my own purposes just as much as he had used me.

My relationship with Hans had been connected to the dynamic with Sam. My father ignored both of us children after the divorce. With unresolved feelings from the loss of his mother, he shut an emotional door on our pain at effectively losing our mother and on the drama of fighting and reconciliation we reenacted in front of his eyes. Raising two kids on his own after being abandoned by his wife burdened Hans in ways I cannot even imagine. And until my brother and I became more independent and mature, Hans closed us out to preserve what was left of his own emotional stability. But the legacy of abandonment left me excessively appreciative of any man, even Sam, who would show me kindness, attention, and love. And in my gratitude and amazement, I disregarded a great deal, including the unhealthy signals Sam had sent.

Ron had his shortcomings too, some evident from the beginning of our courtship and some emerging only later. I never expected to find the perfect partner in him, but I also consciously did not want to repeat the failures of past relationships. I wanted to see Ron for who he was, instead of for what he could give me. And I wanted Ron to see me, deficiencies and all.

For our first wedding anniversary Ron gave me a card. Outside, in large, pink comic-book writing it read, "Who is the best wife in the world?"

"YOU!" was the answer, in huge letters that dominated the front. Below this it asked, "Who's the luckiest spouse in the world?"

Before I opened it, I thought I knew what was written on the inner fold: "Me, your loving husband!" My face spread into a smile. *How sweet*, I thought. He thinks he's lucky to have me.

Instead, when I looked inside the card, there was a reflective piece of plastic in the shape of a large mirror. The card read, "Oh look. It's *you* again!"

I've kept the card, because it sums up Ron and me: both of us acknowledging we're equally lucky to have each other. I learned the importance of reciprocal recognition in part through my experiences with Irmgard. I would come to understand this later even more fully with Hans.

Chapter 19

I'll Always Be with You

2005

Less than two months after my mother died and just at the time
I met Ron, I began attending sessions of a grief group. These
were held at the Unitarian church to which Irmgard had belonged at
the end of her life. In her characteristic style, my mother regarded
the church simply as a social networking system, not as any kind of
religious entity. She volunteered to do clerical work once a month
solely to be allowed to participate in a brown-bag lunch group of re-
tired professional women and to take advantage of other convenient
connections for volunteer opportunities. She never attended Sunday
services and did not set foot in the building except on her office days.

After her death, it seemed natural for me to use her church in
a similar, practical fashion. My search for a grief group began and
ended when I called the same room where my mother had answered
the phone and stuffed envelopes. It was strangely reassuring to think
that, had another daughter called with the same question a year ago,
she could have spoken with Irmgard.

Because the church had received a number of queries similar to
mine in the past months, it planned to start a group to accommodate the requests. Within a few weeks I sat in an upstairs room of the
building with two facilitators and seven other women. Knowing my
mother had spent many hours under the same roof, in the first sessions I felt simultaneously sad and consoled.

All the participants had experienced the loss of a loved one
within the past three years, and all of them, including me, were still
grieving. One woman's daughter had died suddenly almost exactly a

year before, becoming extremely sick while the mother was away in Europe. By the time she had returned to the States, the disease had disfigured her daughter and put her in a coma from which she never emerged. Another woman had lost her partner to illness; another's father had died. Mine was the most recent loss, but a lot of raw, unprocessed emotion swirled around the room.

People don't normally think of "grief group" and "comparison shopping" as fitting together, but I've known a few who have brought that sort of practical appraisal to the process. Pop in to a few sessions here, a few more there. Determine which room or group of people feels like the best fit. Indeed, one might be well advised to do just that.

But I abhorred the idea of quick assessment in the context of my own grief. I knew opening up to my painful emotions would demand more than a little trust. So plunking my heart down in a series of groups to find out where it would be treated with the most compassion and understanding daunted me. I chose the alternative, placing myself at the random mercy of the facilitators and participants in the first group I attended.

DURING THE FIRST EVENING we all sat around a utilitarian, metal conference table in what obviously served as a daycare classroom during business hours. I hardly spoke. When I did, I shared no details about my mother's death. But the facilitators both knew how she had died, because I had participated in an assessment interview before the group began.

I had been honest with them about the events because I wanted to make sure I would not be facing any criticism.

After Irmgard's suicide I felt once again on the defensive, and I could not tolerate the thought that people would judge my memory of her. In my imagination, her death left her more defenseless than she had ever been in life. Only my recollections of her remained. These seemed so vulnerable and my hold on them felt so tenuous that I feared one vehement argument against the rectitude of her decision would turn them to dust in my hand. Because she could no longer model for me her casual indifference to the world's opinion, my fledgling independence cowered inside a hollow shell of bravado, ready to bolt at the first challenge.

During those first months, anything having to do with my mother was an open wound I could not bear anyone to touch. Slowly, I became aware that this disingenuous effort to "protect" Irmgard from being misunderstood put me right back in the position I had been in before I voiced my feelings about her suicide. By avoiding all criticism of her, I prevented myself from speaking the truth about my experience. Feeling entrapped and isolated, I realized my reticence served only to distance me from potential sources of comfort. As I described it during a silent writing exercise that first evening, I felt "dis-abled."

We were to spend five minutes writing about an impersonal object. Looking at a large assortment of random items the facilitators placed in the middle of the square table, I felt drawn to a brooch depicting a woman in a wheelchair. "There is a woman in a wheelchair who is different from other women," I scribbled quickly, without censure. "And the wheelchair is what I think my grief is like. It's different from so many things. It's different from anything I have ever experienced. It distinguishes me from other people in some way. But something separates the experience of the woman on the pin and me. Everyone can look at her and know that she is in a wheelchair and that she's living a life that is different in some ways. But no one can see why I am different, because I am not talking about it."

Grief can be a very isolating ordeal. In part this is due to an almost instinctive need we have to pull into ourselves to heal and regroup. Partially the isolation can be created in reaction to the feedback of others who feel uncomfortable with our situation. But in my case, I also had to acknowledge and liberate myself from the dynamic Irmgard and I had developed, where one person's viewpoint completely obliterated the other's.

IRMGARD AND I HAD prepared for the days immediately following her death as best we could. What to her had originally seemed morbid—"I don't want you to have to think about these kinds of things"—eventually provided us both with a means to feel less overwhelmed. I don't think everyone would have reacted this way, but we were alike enough that we gravitated toward an organizational style of coping. My life immediately after her death became our mutual project. Through working together beforehand on those plans, we created a connection between the two of us that transcended her death. Even after she was gone, I still felt her helping with the onerous duties before me.

With Irmgard's input, I had set up a file on my computer that contained documents entitled "Notify immediately," "Notify at my convenience," "Do first," "Do second," "Do third," and most explicitly, "Upon entering Irmgard's condo for the first time." Looking at this last document now, the comfort we derived from organizing in minute detail what we anticipated would be an excruciating process astonishes me. In part it read:

LIVING ROOM:
    (1) Go to roll-top desk. On the desk there will be unsealed
        letters for me to mail. There will also be a blue folder,
        which contains copies of statements from all accounts,
        with the relevant information highlighted.
    (2) Open the middle drawer of the desk. In there will be:
        (a) information about retirement benefits and pension,
        (b) car title, and
        (c) safe deposit box key.
    (3) In the bottom drawer of the desk are checkbooks, which,
        as a co-signer, I can use for funeral and other expenses.

Despite our advance planning, in those first weeks my duties sometimes overwhelmed me. At times I had the landline telephone receiver to one ear, the cell phone to the other, and call waiting beeping on each. Although the pain of not having Irmgard around gnawed fiercely at my heart, I also derived comfort from still being needed by her. I found gratification in making her final, post-death impression on the world one of organization, minimalism, and dignity.

After the external trappings of my world returned to their normal routine, grief settled in as my quiet but painful companion. I had the usual symptoms—crying at inopportune moments and being sentimentally moved by the smallest details. I suffered a physical pain relentlessly present in the middle of my chest. *So this is heartache?* I rubbed my ribs often, trying to alleviate the discomfort. Although certainly a physical sensation, it did not dissipate with any amount of massage. It stayed with me for weeks.

Nevertheless, I considered myself to be coping well. My pre-death grieving had intruded more on my work and my daily routine than the post-death grieving did. I also had a sense of having experienced the miraculous. I had emerged alive from underneath the train that had run me over. I had survived the horrible and long-dreaded experience. Along with the pain of loss came incredible relief that the worst was over. I felt a new faith in my own inner strength for having borne the unbearable.

I joined the grief group in the spring after Irmgard's death more as a failsafe than out of a desperate need.

"I think I'm doing fine in general," I explained during the assessment interview, "but I want to be certain I'm not ignoring some part of me that's not."

What I learned in the group was that I was right on both counts. I coped well. But I also hid unexpressed pain, and I benefited from exploring more of my thinking and grieving processes.

In an imagined dialogue with my mother during the fourth class, I wrote as if Irmgard were asking me questions:

Irmgard: "Tina, how are you?"
Me: "I'm okay. In the beginning this was so much harder
    than either of us ever imagined it would be. Do you hear
    that? It was harder, in the beginning, than anything I've
    ever experienced, times ten. I want you to know how
    much I suffered because of what you did."

Irmgard: "I hear you. How can I help you now?"

Me: "Well, it's not really you who can help, but there is one thing that I still feel very tied to. I would like to come to more peace about selling your condo, since it is a place you loved so much. You said goodbye to it, and you knew I was going to sell it. I won't be the only person who has closed that door, never to come back. But I always thought that you were the one who was so obsessed with protecting me from everything. Now I see that I was really obsessed with protecting you. I'm doing it even after you're gone, when you can't possibly care anymore. You can't care about the condo. And if you don't care, then what I'm experiencing is really about me."

Irmgard: "Tina, you know that I always wanted you to be happy."

Me: "I know. And I'm trying to come to terms with your death. So . . . let me just ask. Is it okay with you that I sell the condo?"

Irmgard: "Yes! Of course! I loved it. You liked it. But you have your own house. The condo made me very, very happy to come home to every day. If you find a place that you are happy to come home to every day, I will be happiest. I want you to know the contentment I had."

Without the group, I don't know whether I would have been able to come to that conclusion. Or to others like it.

Eventually, I did tell the members how my mother had died. Their nonjudgmental reaction and support created the first hole in the armor I used to shield my memory of Irmgard. That armor took a very long time to disintegrate, but awareness was the first step. *Hello, my name is Tina, and I'm protecting my mother's memory.*

Next, or maybe this came first, stories from other members about their losses helped me. Their accounts gave my reactions a context and a voice. Even if I experienced things differently, the group discussion and the leaders' input made my response part of a universal process. My previously disjointed emotions took on substance and heft. More and more I realized that in some fashion Irmgard and I had been extremely fortunate. Knowing the date of her death, we had taken advantage of the time we had left to communicate with increasing openness. Of course, Irmgard's giving me a twenty-year head start to think about her loss felt unnecessary and cruel. Nevertheless, she and I parted with no unfulfilled wishes. We left no final words unspoken. We tried to think of everything we wanted to say, or do, or feel, and anything that we forgot, such as the condo, could be understood in retrospect.

It took me longer to understand that my wholehearted acceptance of Irmgard's "my way or the highway" attitude regarding her suicide had affected not only me.

Chapter 20

What's It All About?

2005, 2006, 2007

The shackles Irmgard placed on me, I in turn clamped on others. Before her death, when I told someone of my mother's plans, my manner made it tacitly clear: I would tolerate no disagreement. Even after her suicide, I abided nothing less.

But through the introspection the grief group engendered, I learned more about my own complicity in the psychologically damaging interplay between the two of us. Still, I began to grasp the magnitude of my self-delusion only when Lucy declared, "Tina, you say your mother was sadistic. But you should take a good look at yourself!"

After Irmgard's death, I had gradually noticed a change in my relationship with my best friend. I observed only subtle differences at first, things I discounted without much reflection. Progressively, the signs became more obvious: a cold response to an invitation to visit, long descriptions of the gifts she bought for others' birthdays and not even a card to acknowledge mine. She didn't commit grand, friendship-breaking offenses, but I noted them with increasing apprehension.

Finally, her attitude toward me became openly hostile, but instead of addressing the rift head-on, I retreated, baffled and scared. I had no clear idea why she was acting in that way. And yet, in the fog of my bewilderment, one isolated thought intermittently nudged its way into my consciousness: *This has something to do with Irmgard.* From hints Lucy had dropped, from things she had left unsaid, I intimated that she might be angry with my mother.

When we finally spoke about our problems openly, she informed me Irmgard had not angered her. *I* had.

She had never approved of my mother's plans, yet I had never given her the leeway in our relationship to express anything counter to Irmgard's party line. She went along with it but felt continually oppressed because she had to choose between maintaining our friendship and revealing her true feelings. And now with Irmgard dead, Lucy honestly feared that someday I would kill myself too. She agonized that I would repeat the cycle, taking my life and giving her no say in the matter. Our friendship would not be considered; no disagreement would be tolerated.

My mother put a gag in my mouth, and I put one in my best friend's.

My way or the highway. What a chilling concept. No room for argument. No room for love. No gentle dissuasion or compromise. Just a dictatorship in which all dissidents are exiled.

Except I had learned more than one thing from Irmgard. She had taught me how to lay down the law, but she had also taught me what it felt like to be punished. When Lucy finally expressed how she had suffered, the fury flaring in her eyes, for the first time I truly perceived the insidious baggage my family had handed down from generation to generation. My grandparents had passed something ice cold and desperate to my mother, and she had transferred that same burden to me.

I held Lucy's gaze, and although my heart ached at the thought of what I had done to her, I moved toward her rage. "I don't think I can ever apologize enough, Lucy. I am *not* going to do what my mother did, not now, and not in the future. But I can see why you thought that, and I'm terribly sorry." I halted, searching for an adequate summation. "Your opinion and the opinions of the other people I love matter to me a great deal. And I promise you I will live the rest of my life taking them into account."

My words inadequately expressed my sentiments, but Lucy accepted my apology. She understood.

THE SIX MONTHS FOLLOWING my mother's death in February 2005 exemplified Nietzsche's pronouncement, "What does not kill me, makes me stronger." I felt prepared for anything.

And then it happened. Hans had his massive stroke, and I began the gradual slide back toward darkness.

It did seem strange to me that after his stroke, I didn't cry about losing Hans to dementia. I cried more often and more deeply about losing my mother. Ron would come into the bedroom after we'd spent a day at the nursing home and find me curled up on the bed in the dark, cradling in my hands a photo of my mother from the last day I saw her. I wept so hard that the pillow had to be dried out.

"I miss her so much," I would sob yet again.

In my rational moments, none of this made much sense to me. Why, upon watching my father ripped from sentient life, did I grieve for Irmgard so? Why didn't I dream of Hans's arms around me or hear his comforting words in my ears?

This was the one thing neither Irmgard nor I had planned for. We had anticipated so much else, but that I would need her so desperately, so soon after her death, we never once considered.

If we had known ahead of time, I know what she would have done. We never discussed it, but I know with conviction that she would not have let me suffer the aftermath of Hans's incapacitation alone had there been a warning. Had she known Hans would become completely incapacitated in late 2005, she would have changed her plans for killing herself early that same year. She would have postponed her death. Perhaps only for another year, until I had my bearings, but she would have done it. Not for Hans, but for me.

I knew this, and I cried for our not having had the choice to make. I cried for my being left alone to deal with things that would have been so much easier if shared with her. Now, for the first time, I understood the type of loss that had been discussed in the grief group. The loss contingent upon, "I wish I had . . ." For I wished desperately, not for my father to return to himself, which I knew was impossible, but for an even more unrealistic and barbaric fantasy: I wished for my father's stroke to have happened earlier.

It's not that I loved my father less. Rather, deserted by both parents within the course of six months, I wished to rearrange history and create a scenario to help me avoid some of the pain. If both parents had to leave me permanently, at least there could have been a better order, I rationalized. Suffer the unexpected before the expected. Deal with the shock and grief and burden of caring for my impaired father before the more orderly and prepared-for death of my mother.

That is the way I secretly wished it had gone. But of course it happened differently.

A PROFESSOR IN SOCIAL work school once told my class, "Everything is about loss, and so everything is really about death." Not exactly uplifting, but this was, after all, a class in clinical psychology, and he was referring to the issues brought up by clients in therapy sessions.

For me his words ring true far beyond the classroom or the couch. Death is the only inevitable loss all human beings recognize. So it makes sense that most of our fear, anger, sadness, jealousy, and anxiety consciously or unconsciously revolve around that central, immutable truth. In essence, the smaller losses in life manifest diminutive versions of the gargantuan elephant that's always lurking in the collective human living room. What we believe happens to us after our organs cease to function, and how strongly we hold to this belief, may mitigate or accentuate our feelings about death. But no matter what we believe, the end of our time on earth will come. And for most of us, it comes on its own schedule.

Hans's third hemorrhagic stroke took place in July 2006, approximately a year after his first. It happened on a Friday and was nearly as large as his second. Everyone I met predicted Hans would not live through the weekend. The nursing home staff found Hans "unresponsive" in his bed at the five a.m. check. Against the orders in his chart, they called an ambulance to take him to the emergency room of the nearest hospital.

In keeping with the unpredictable malfunctioning of the blood vessels in his brain, this third stroke had nothing to do with the previous two. It occurred in a completely different location, above his brain stem. But the doctors again made dire predictions. The eagerness with which the young attending physician jumped at my question about hospice care unnerved me.

"So you're telling me the blood will probably clot and block the exit pathway for other fluid to leave his brain. That doesn't sound good," I said.

"Well . . ." the doctor hesitated, "we really just have to wait and see what happens."

His answer seemed to be avoiding some central questions, and I wanted concrete information about what to do. Hans couldn't stay in the emergency room forever. "Should he be hospitalized?"

Awkward silence.

I forged along, heeding the words he left unspoken. "Should I try and get him into hospice?"

"Hospice. Yes! That's a really good idea." The doctor's face suddenly brightened.

"Okay," I said, slightly taken aback, "but I have no idea how to go about that. Do I just call some number?"

"Don't worry," he said, clasping his hands together. "I'll make a phone call for you." He paused and added, "We should try to get him enrolled this weekend, so they can start coming." Hospice in Delaware meant that hospice workers would visit the nursing home, not that Hans would be transferred to another facility.

Afterward, I learned from the staff that my father had returned from the hospital with papers indicating he was not expected to live through the night, to say nothing of the weekend. Perhaps that explains why, to my great surprise, he officially became a hospice patient by six o'clock the very same evening. What I first regarded as extreme efficiency I should probably have attributed to the emergency room doctor's phrasing to the hospice intake nurse— something like "not likely to live more than twenty-four hours" got the paperwork moving.

As usual, however, all predictions about Hans were wrong. Not only did he live through the weekend, but he lived long enough to be thrown out of yet another program. Months passed after the stroke.

Hans's speech and mobility improved, he ate and drank by himself again, and eventually I got calls from the hospice social worker that they no longer considered him eligible for hospice care. After all, the admission criteria specified that someone must have a life expectancy of six months or less, and Hans no longer looked moribund. As a matter of fact, he had gained ten pounds. I lobbied for him, citing studies showing that the likelihood of a subsequent hemorrhage after multiple occurrences is very high and other studies indicating that minimally enhanced physical functioning does not equate with longer life expectancy. I gained him another month of care. But in the end he was again kicked out, this time for the decidedly non-aggressive behavior of continuing to thrive.

During hospice care, Hans's doctor had discontinued his remaining medications. Hans had been rather highly medicated at the Quaker Community because of his aggressive behaviors, and the nursing home had continued administering the existing regimen. Since hospice treatment is designed around palliative care, it left Hans with only skin cream and some pills for constipation. It turned out he would not have needed to continue taking the antipsychotics and antidepressants anyway, because, yet again, this latest stroke had also affected his personality. Miraculously, it changed him for the better. More connections in his brain died, and *voilà!*—he became more docile. He still screamed, but his cries now expressed genuine frustration or discomfort, not fury directed toward specific individuals. He no longer threatened the staff, verbally or physically, and although he could sometimes deliver a completely on-target ironic remark, the malicious intent had disappeared.

After this stroke Hans experienced a distinct yet gradual decline in his cognitive abilities, but if viewed on a graph, the downward trend would have been punctuated by many peaks and valleys. The personality of the former Hans still existed, but only in attenuated form. His dementia steadily eroded his memory. Toward the end, he only recognized with consistency his children and their spouses.

Strangely, the subtler aspects of his personality often emerged unexpectedly. Sometimes he responded to a conversation with a sentence that let you know he still had a good idea of your basic character. And sometimes a simple gesture or look enabled you to project the old Hans onto the new.

As for inhibitions, he had very few. If he was constipated, the discomfort of feeling stopped up made him very vocal. If his skin got pinched or his arm fell asleep, he yelled at the top of his lungs. He dozed during conversations. But he did not shy away from laughing and crying or making jokes. It made me question my own self-consciousness, which sometimes held me back from expressing myself.

ALTOGETHER, HANS LED A tolerable life in those years.

He lived in a facility where the staff treated him with kindness and dignity. I never announced my visits, and neither did my brother, and yet we never saw anything disturbing, even in the evenings or on weekends. Hans's brother, Walter, came to visit, staying in a hotel nearby for a week, and he confirmed the sense we had. After spending eight to twelve hours a day with my father during all the nursing shifts, he returned to Germany with a very favorable impression.

Of course, I had not chosen the facility by accident. In the search for a new home for Hans after the Quaker Community, I toured ten facilities and spoke by phone with many more. I created an extended checklist of questions, which I put together based on information from journal articles, websites, and consultations with nursing home staff. Weathering annoyed looks, I persistently queried directors about the number of registered nurses on every shift and the ratio of nurse aides to residents. I asked to see copies of the latest inspection reports and questioned staff about turnover rates. I selected the new nursing home not because of its beauty but because of its high-quality care and its resident-centered philosophy.

But Hans had certainly hoped for a better end to his life.

He and I talked about this. I sometimes had difficulty holding a conversation with him, because the quality of the discussions depended on his mood, physical comfort, and mental alertness, as well as the degree of environmental distraction. Despite these challenges, especially in the weeks after the third stroke when everyone was still certain Hans would not live long, I often broached the subject of death.

I have videos of some of those startling conversations. Although they were punctuated by long silences and intervals of frustration as Hans searched for a word, he spoke with remarkable lucidity. During one of those halting talks, when I told him I would try my best to be there with him when he died, he replied: "Tina, . . . I appreciate that. But . . . it doesn't . . . it doesn't really . . . matter. I have . . . to . . . walk . . . through . . . that door by myself . . . But . . . I'm not ready . . . to open . . . it . . . yet."

That was how he had felt about death before the stroke. Some things had not changed.

His photo stood in many places around my home and office. The Hans looking at me in these pictures was the loving father I once had. The man who sat in the wheelchair when I visited the nursing home still loved me, but I tried hard not to expect anything of him. Yet sometimes I reacted strongly to his actions or emotions, especially to his sadness. For while he now perceived all his losses as transitory events, perhaps to be revisited soon but always new when they reappeared, the experience of his pain lingered with me.

Chapter 21

Comfort Measures

2008

At three in the afternoon on December 26, 2008, I sat alone in my study in Massachusetts. The president had declared this day after Christmas a federal holiday. He may have envisioned people engaging in economy-boosting, post-party shopping sprees, but I contentedly spent my time indoors, reveling at the prospect of a long weekend with nothing in particular on the agenda. Snow from a massive, nineteen-inch fall less than a week earlier still blanketed the ground outside my second-story window. I could look out over our short driveway and the street beyond to the neighbors' manicured hedges trimmed with diminutive crowns of white.

I snuggled down in my father's old lounge chair. With my shiny new computer on my lap, I leaned back and talked to Lucy over the Internet. On the screen, her face in Germany appeared tired, and she struggled to find a position in her bed across the ocean that allowed her to relax. We had only had a video chat once before, and despite the late hour for her, the experience still enthralled us.

When the telephone's ring interrupted our conversation, I ignored it. Ron was downstairs in his study, and I assumed one of his Seattle friends was calling after lunch on the West Coast. When he came upstairs and knocked on my door, I felt no twinge. When Ron poked his head inside, holding the cordless phone receiver and telling me, "It's the nursing home on the phone. They have some news about your father," none of my senses jingled in anticipatory fear. *It's probably just someone asking me to buy him some extra socks,* I thought.

"Lucy, I'll call you back. This won't take long," I said, before replacing the laptop on the desk, standing up, and walking the short distance to the door.

"Hello?" I said when Ron handed me the receiver.

"Hello, Tina? This is Cheryl, the nurse at the nursing home. Honey, I just came on my shift, and I want you to know that there's been a change in your father's condition. Tina, he doesn't look good. I don't know how long he's been like this. The nurse who was on before said he had some 'gurgling' in his lungs. But honey, that's no gurgling. I listened. He's aspirated. It said in the chart that he had the stomach flu yesterday. It's been going around the whole nursing home. He was vomiting and had diarrhea for twenty minutes straight. And it's possible that he aspirated his own vomit."

All thoughts drained from my mind, leaving only a single sentence: *This might be it.*

I had taken the phone into our bedroom. In my shock, I focused on the cat, curled up in a perfect circle, creating a brown-and-black-striped indentation in the pink comforter cover. Looking at the calmly sleeping animal, I sat on the corner of the bed as I slowly assimilated the nurse's words. "Okay. So . . . aspiration." I thought about the things I knew about how older people die. "The next thing would be to expect pneumonia, right?"

"That's right. That could happen. Now, I know it says here in the chart not to hospitalize him."

"Absolutely. That's correct. Don't hospitalize him." I thought about Irmgard and how Hans's increasingly dependent and impaired state was exactly the fate she had wanted to avoid. I felt certain that Hans would not want to prolong things either, if destiny was now intervening.

"Okay. I understand. I just wanted to make sure. I have him on oxygen. But I have to tell you, he doesn't look good."

"Will you keep me informed if there's any change?"

"I will keep checking on him, and if there's a change, I'll call you back right away."

"Thank you. Thank you very much for that. I might call you back, too."

"That's fine, honey. You call back anytime. I just wanted to let you know."

I hung up.

This did not sound like a false alarm. I knew that pneumonia in the elderly, even *with* treatment, can be life threatening. My emotional antennae had risen to full alert, and I felt as though I had just drunk four cups of coffee.

Before going downstairs to talk with Ron, before getting back online with Lucy, I returned to my study and picked up my father's living will. I had found it during my recent basement cleanup, at the same time I had found the documentation of my parents' early years.

Hans's living will clearly affirmed his wishes. "Were I to become terminally ill with little expectation of recovering from severe mental or physical disability," it read, "I request that comfort measures take priority over the use of heroic medical measures which would prolong the dying process. . . . Decisions about withholding and/or withdrawing life support treatments may take place very rapidly. . . . I wish to acknowledge my deep gratitude to caregivers, family, and friends for assisting in honoring these directives, and by doing so, allowing me in my dying another opportunity for spiritual growth." A bit New Age in its wording, it nevertheless proclaimed some frank directives.

I called Lucy back, and we discussed the sudden change in Hans's condition. We talked about my having anticipated the arrival of this moment for the past three years, and she gave voice to feelings she rightly expected me to have.

"I can imagine that a part of you must be relieved Hans's suffering is going to end," she guessed.

Without warning, tears welled up in my eyes. Abruptly faced with the imminent prospect of my father's death, I did not feel relieved. I could not do anything but accept what would happen. I could not take sides and hope for one outcome over another. And it gave me no joy that I would be helping his death along by enacting his wish to refrain from hospitalization and intravenous antibiotics. Instead of my usual role of primary actor in the drama of my father's life, at that moment I desperately would have preferred a seat in the audience.

IN THE PREVIOUS YEARS I had often thought about what Hans's memorial celebration would be like. People must do this all the time, hold ceremonies for loved ones whose last years of life were not in any way similar to the bulk of their time on this planet. I wondered who came to those events, and what people remembered when they went.

It was strange to think about such a service for my father. So many of his friends were older than he. By the time my father's body gave out, some of his friends' bodies would have beaten his to it. For those still alive, how many would attend? And who would they be coming for? Hans as he was at the end, or the Hans they used to know?

Some of his acquaintances probably did not realize Hans had not simply grown tired of their relationship or inconsiderately let contact slip away. There may even have been a person or two who harbored residual anger at my father for his role in the silence between them. Admittedly, I did not systematically go through Hans's address book and call everyone. I did not write to them and tell them where he was and how his life had changed.

In thinking about his death, I had anticipated and even hoped for a number of things for Hans. A sudden fatal heart attack caused by his deliberately untreated high cholesterol and unrestrained love of sweets. A final hemorrhagic stroke precipitated by the damage inflicted during his previous three. An undefined physical malfunction related to his age or genetic characteristics that quickly and painlessly robbed him of his life. But in all my musings I had not anticipated death-by-stomach-flu.

I called Cheryl back.

"Look, I know I said not to hospitalize him. But I really want to be clear. No antibiotics. No drastic measures. Nothing."

"I understand. I faxed the doctor about his condition, but that's all I did. It's all clear. If it comes to it, comfort measures only."

"Yes, comfort measures. Please make him as comfortable as possible."

After speaking again with Cheryl, I needed to get out of the house and think about what might be coming. I put on my tallest snow boots and walked north on the bike path behind our house toward the small local lake. I crunched through the snow, alone in the stillness of the trail.

Deep gratitude for assisting in honoring these directives. I repeated those words from the living will to myself as I tried to envision Hans walking along beside me. It was difficult to concentrate my senses on imagining his large, strong hand gripping mine. The image of him remained for only a few seconds before I was distracted by a patch of ice on the path, difficult to see in the twilight. Nevertheless, I tried to ask him what I should do. Whether I was doing the right thing.

"No antibiotics, right? That's what you want, right?"

My ephemeral vision of him never stayed around long enough to give me an answer.

At the lake I looked out over the recently frozen black surface. A sliver of a moon gave off hardly any light in the clear sky, and stars and planets began to twinkle. I stood amid fallen trees, toppled into the lake by beavers. The trees lay around the edge, stripped naked of their bark, creating a series of slides into the water. I tried to imagine their branches' invisible, interlacing network of hiding places below the surface.

Lucy and I had seen a beaver quite near this spot in the fall. Its head had poked suddenly out of the water and looked around. We both held our breath and stood frozen, not wanting to alert it to our presence. The tiny eyes scanned the surroundings for a few moments before it lazily dived down, its glistening brown back and then its long, flat tail disappearing with scarcely a ripple into the submerged tangle of limbs.

This evening, however, peace reigned absolute.

"No antibiotics?" I called quietly across the water.

Still no answer, except a rapid rustle as a sudden gust of wind shook old leaves in the trees around me.

"Okay. No antibiotics," I declared to the moon and turned my back on the lake to head home.

IT SEEMED TO ME that I had only just entered the kitchen when the phone rang again. Ron came into the room. I looked at him with foreboding before I reached for the receiver. It was Cheryl.

"Tina? Honey, I'm really sorry to call. And I don't usually say this. But honey, I don't think he's going to make it through the night."

"He's gotten worse?"

"Yes. I can't believe how much he's deteriorated since I came on my shift. I'm going to take the cordless phone into his room and sit by him so that I can keep an eye on him. I don't want him to be alone."

"Okay. Thank you. I appreciate that." I paused. I couldn't think. My mind emptied, save for a single command: *Go!*

"I think I'm going to try to get down there," I told her.

I turned to Ron after hanging up. "I've got to go. The car's in the shop. What do we do?"

His face melted into kindness. "Tina, I'm so sorry. I know you want me to go with you. But I really think it would be faster if you flew. I'll get the car tomorrow and drive down if you need me."

Fly. Of course.

WAITING AT THE AIRPORT gate, I called a few of my father's old friends. I wanted to share the news, and I also wanted to give them a warning about what to expect. *Better to call now*, I reasoned, *at a decent hour, than to be torn about whether or not to wake them up in the middle of the night if worse comes to worst.* But I also did not want to be in this alone anymore. I wanted people's thoughts to be with me during the next hours. Hearing their comforting voices moved me to the tears I had not been able to release before.

Not surprisingly, not a single rental car was available at the Philadelphia airport the day after Christmas. No minivan, no economy-size two-door, no SUV, no luxury sedan—nothing could I rent at this busy metropolitan airway hub. With a growing sense of panic I imagined the vast emptiness of the rental company parking lots. *How will I get to the nursing home?*

My fear only lasted until I reminded myself I did not have to do everything alone. Even though I still instinctually gravitated toward independent action, I had also developed a new skill in the past three years: the ability to lean on other people. *Call your friends. Somebody can come to the airport and drive you there.* People could support me. Isolation no longer had to be my standard operating procedure.

And so the inefficiency of the rental car companies forced me to start the final journey to see my father much differently from the way the last few years with him had begun. On this visit I was never alone.

Chris, the wife of my ex-husband's only brother, picked me up. During my years married to Sam, Chris and I had become the most intimate of confidants; only she understood from an insider's perspective just how trapped and miserable I felt in the marriage. After the divorce, I remained close to her family. That evening, after getting my desperate phone call, Chris had ditched the clan's annual Christmas festivities to come get me.

We entered the darkened nursing home building at eleven. A Christmas tree lit the entrance. Dense silver and gold ornamentation adorned it, and I could hardly discern the green plastic twigs holding the decorations aloft. Its exuberant display seemed gratingly incongruent with our mission. From the ceiling of the first-floor hallway hung colorful glass balls of purple and gold in addition to sparkling snowflake cutouts. Someone had spaced these in regular intervals and suspended them high enough to remain out of the reach of even the most determined resident. We entered the elevator, our hearts racing in anticipation of what we would find, and the doors closed slowly behind us.

Immediately upon stepping out at the second floor, we heard a racket I took to be my father's oxygen machine: loud bubbling in constant intervals. It sounded like the noise made when sucking the last of a milkshake from the bottom of a glass through a straw. Only exponentially louder.

Upon entering Hans's room, I realized the sound was not mechanical. It emanated from my father's lungs. Over the distressing reverberations in his chest you couldn't even hear the oxygen machine pumping at full capacity. "Respirations rapid and labored with audible crackling," the nurse had noted in his chart.

He was in agony. He was essentially asphyxiating. And he was terrified.

Although he took four breaths for every one of mine, Hans couldn't manage to get enough air, despite the oxygen mask. With dramatic diaphragmatic inhalation, his chest expanded and contracted more than I ever imagined was physically possible. His abdomen looked like a basketball constantly being deflated and blown up again. The sheer energy involved in sustaining that type of breathing would have exhausted even the healthiest individual. And Hans had been keeping this up for hours already.

Nevertheless, Hans reacted to my arrival. When I told him I was there, his gasps became more intense and his reactions more alert. I moved to the side of the bed and stroked his hand. He reached for mine, albeit slowly, and crushed it in his grip. I didn't realize he had so much strength left. Although contorted in his never-ending quest for more oxygen, his face radiated fright.

A nurse entered the room. Shifts had changed hours earlier, and Nurse Cheryl was gone. From Hans's bedside I spoke with the new person. "He's suffering. And I don't think it's necessary. If he needs to be on hospice to get some relief, I'll make the call right now. Just tell me what I need to do. We have to do something to stop this. He needs morphine or something to ease what he's going through."

She looked at him for a few moments and then agreed to call the doctor. Knowing Hans would be relying on her, I chose not to mention she should have done this a while ago.

Chris sat in a recliner. I pulled a straight-backed chair up to the free side of Hans's bed, reaching awkwardly across his body to hold his right hand. With my left hand I stroked his face while I spoke to him.

"Hans, let me tell you what is going on. You have pneumonia.

You . . ." And then I stopped as I remembered it might be easier for him to understand if I put the entire situation into context. "You have had a number of severe hemorrhagic strokes," I began my monologue again. "You have been in a nursing home for over three years. It hasn't been easy for you, but they have taken good care of you. Now yesterday you had the stomach flu, and you vomited a lot. I think you aspirated some of your own vomit. That means it got into your lungs, and it's causing an infection. That's why it's so hard for you to breathe now.

"I read your living will again, Hans. You might not remember. You wrote it a long time ago. It said that you do not want drastic measures taken to prolong your life. So now I am going to follow your wishes. You are not going to be hospitalized. You are not going to get antibiotics. And that means that you are going to die. There's no question this time."

I repeated the next words slowly. "You are going to die, but I *am going to make sure* your suffering ends. You are going to get morphine. Your breathing is going to get easier. Don't worry. The distress you feel won't last much longer.

"I know you're really scared and this is really uncomfortable for you now. Try and relax." I wanted to tell him to take a deep breath, as I often had when he had been worked up in the past. But luckily I stopped myself in time. *He is taking deep breaths.*

"Think about all the good things in your life, Hans," I continued. "You had a very good life. You really had a lot of fun. When all of your family went back to East Germany, you forged yourself a new life by coming to the U.S. You embraced everything here. You made new friends. You got a PhD. You got married and had two children. You raised us. You developed your hobbies. Your friends really love you, and you were a great help to them. You were an inspiration to many people. And your son and daughter love you very much."

Thinking my soliloquy finished, I took my gaze from his wide eyes. Then I remembered what the hospice nurse had told me two years before, that dying people often hang on because they think others need them. So I hastily added, as though it were not an afterthought, "But we will be okay after you die. Don't worry about us. We will never forget you. You will live on in our hearts, and we'll be fine." And, even though I didn't want to lie, I tried to reassure him on an existential level as well. I added, "And don't worry about death. It's going to be okay."

At various times during my speech, Hans wrinkled his face. I recognized the expression. If he had been able to breathe properly, he would have begun to cry. He was not at peace with the prospect of his own death. It might have been easier for me if he had nodded tranquilly at my telling him his life would undeniably end soon. It might have been easier, but it would not have been consistent with who he was. He was not my mother, going quietly, calmly about the choice she had made. Nothing in the last three years of Hans's life had been his choice. It wasn't his choice to have everything end now. Nevertheless, I was not sure how much of his disquiet was unavoidable because of his own personality and unfulfilled desires, and how much of it was due to the harrowing circumstances in which he found himself. Fighting for air as though he were a goldfish unmercifully plucked from its bowl, he would have had to muster something more than courage to achieve peace of mind.

This was why he needed morphine. It would help relieve his mental anguish in addition to calming some of his symptoms. If his struggle had to continue, I could at least ensure that it was devoid of pain and conscious participation.

Unfortunately for Hans, in this age of mail-order pharmacies, it took until two in the morning for his morphine to arrive. Every half hour or so, Chris and I would look at the clock. Chris would leave to search for the nurse while Hans continued to squeeze my hand. Having to cover all three floors of the facility by herself, the night shift nurse sometimes proved difficult to find. When she arrived, she invariably agreed he was not getting any better. But until the medication arrived, she said she could not do much else.

While waiting, I stroked my father's rough, feverish brow. I wet a paper towel and ran it over his thin lips, removing some of the sticky, congealed saliva that had accumulated on them. He was not able to drink and was becoming severely dehydrated. He had anticipated this, too, in his living will, stating he was "aware that dehydration can be uncomfortable, [but that he believed] in trusting the wisdom of the body." I ran the moistened paper towel inside his dentureless mouth, feeling the breeze of his gasping breaths on my hand. *Trusting the wisdom of the body.* When he had written those six words, I wondered whether Hans had actually seen someone die of dehydration, fever, and a raging bacterial infection.

This was certainly new territory for me. My father lay in front of me, dying, and I wanted everything he experienced from me to convey the depth of my love. But I imagine that the situation must be similar to having a child get sick. You love your child, and the child has done nothing deliberately, but sometimes the tasks you must undertake disturb you. It has nothing to do with the *who* but with the *what*.

The smell and feel of Hans bothered me. The breath from his open mouth was rank, the skin on his forehead was bumpy and rough, and his age-defying blond hair glistened with sweat from his fever. His untrimmed fingernails clawed into my skin when he gripped my hand tightly.

He couldn't help any of this, of course. If he had been able to shower, he would have. Shower, shave, clip his nails. *The time for that is over*, I reminded myself. And I knew my gestures were the last ones Hans would feel before losing awareness forever. So I pulled myself together, ignored my reactions to the what, and concentrated instead on the who.

Just as with my mother in her last days, those final hours with Hans no longer allowed any room for "Tina" in the communication between us. I had not expected this parallel between the situations. My mother had died so differently. Yet for me, left behind in both cases, the circumstances felt eerily similar. I focused now on Hans, the person for whom there was going to be no tomorrow. Everything had to be all about what he needed to make his process easier. About what I could do for him. Everything was all about him.

Or so I thought.

Chapter 22

A Different Final Exit

2008

I spent the rest of the night at Hans's side, either touching his arm or just sitting facing him. The sound of his panting kept me awake. I feared if I fell asleep and his respirations became more distressed, I might not notice. And if I dozed and his breathing stopped, I also might not notice. Both ideas supplied my nervous system with a continual influx of adrenaline. It wasn't difficult to stay awake; it was difficult to imagine sleeping. And so I kept vigil. And every time Hans started to become the slightest bit aware of his surroundings, I quietly got up and found the nurse and had her administer another dose of morphine.

At three in the morning at my father's bedside, I twisted around in my chair to face Chris. I asked the question that had been plaguing my mind since our arrival four hours earlier: "When are you going to leave, Chris?"

Her matter-of-fact answer took me completely off guard. "I'm not," she said. "You don't want me to leave, do you?"

"No."

"Then I'm staying until you tell me to go. I can't imagine leaving you alone in a situation like this." And after a pause she added, "I know you'd do the same for me."

I nodded with relief and turned back to Hans.

That night I did not lack for companions. Chris curled up in the armchair, fitfully sleeping for a few hours. And across the opening of my father's door passed mute images of nocturnal nursing home activity. An older man shuffled rapidly by at regular intervals, like a metronome, intent on fulfilling some inexplicable mission. His upper back was bent, so that his graying head faced the floor, unaware of the world around him. At either end of the hallway, he seemingly became disgruntled with his attire. He first passed wearing a navy fleece bathrobe. Then at the next viewing the wrap was slung around his shoulders. Sometimes his shuffling feet, which seemed desperate to catch up with each other in a race to an unknown goal, were clad in red felt slippers. At other times he had on only white gym socks. Later still he had changed out of his striped flannel pajama pants entirely and wore only the robe again. He carried the pajamas on his bent arm as he whizzed by, like a valet proffering pressed trousers.

I also noticed the woman in the pink housecoat, who peeked into our room with a wrinkled brow and troubled eyes. She always stood at the threshold with her mouth pursed in a sour expression, as though she wanted to come in but at the last minute noticed something distasteful that kept her away.

The presence of these insomniacs neither disturbed nor comforted me. Along with the sleeping residents and my dying father, they represented old age in its range of possibilities. They were my father's cohort, with only history and genetics, accident and illness separating one from another.

The day shift arrived before seven in the morning, and with more staff on hand, the morphine doses and the periodic changing of Hans's position became regular. The day nurse assured me that Hans would not die within the next hour. She encouraged Chris and me to go out for a quick breakfast. It felt surreal to step into the refreshing air after a night of cloistered calamity.

In the afternoon, after thirty hours without sleep, I finally left Hans's side for more than a brief interval. My brother, Warner, arrived. He would stay until early evening. Ron's sister picked me up for a few hours of sleep at her house before another all-night shift.

Two hours later she was driving me back to the nursing home.

"I've never been so happy to see lighted reindeer on people's lawns!" she exclaimed as she used the leftover Christmas decorations to navigate through the dense fog that had settled on the elevated land outside of town. She lowered her speed and concentrated on plotting a course based on inflated Santas, trees strung with lights, and glowing animals. It seemed unnaturally welcoming when, as we entered town, the fog suddenly dissipated.

In the end, Hans's death had turned out to be a non-event. In contrast to his dramatic suffering, two hours after I had left his bedside Hans had simply stopped breathing when his brain no longer received enough oxygen to function. Never having seen a dead body before, I was nervous as I stepped out of the elevator onto the second floor again. But I needn't have been. Detached from the machines, Hans lay in the unusual stillness of the room, finally at peace. The nurses had closed his eyes and placed his hands on his chest, a relaxed pose showing none of the struggle that had preceded it.

Looking at Hans's face, I had difficulty not continually imagining that his torso moved in a slight intake of breath. Then when I stared at his chest to reassure myself the nurse had not made an error, out of the corner of my eye I could have sworn his nostrils flared. My eyes flashed back and forth countless times until I convinced myself he was gone. I laid my hands on his and kissed his still-warm cheek one last time.

Shortly afterward, the veteran nurse on duty tried to pull me out of the room. The funeral home staff had arrived, pushing an empty body bag on a stretcher. "Trust me," she urged. "You *really* don't need to see this. They're bringing him out in a *bag*. I've been here thirty years and I still don't like to see it."

"Don't worry," I responded, astonished by her vehemence. "It's just a body. I'm fine."

I didn't mind seeing them wheel the stretcher down the hallway. The bag and the stretcher were both an attractive, subdued maroon, not the sterile black I had seen in movies. The two men, one clean-cut in his twenties and the other older and more rotund, both wore dark suits. They moved with the utmost solemnity. I had no doubt they would treat my father with respect.

After they left and I had completed all the paperwork, I stepped back into Hans's room for one last look around. Everything seemed the same. And yet everything had changed.

FOR MORE THAN THREE years, every answering machine message, every missed call, every telephone ring in the middle of the night—none had gone unchecked or unanswered. If I had company when the phone rang, I simply excused myself for a moment. I moved an extra extension next to my side of the bed. I had my cell phone turned on and with me at all times. Because from the moment the downstairs neighbor went to check on Hans in September 2005, I had been waiting. A coil had been wound tightly inside me, ready to spring into action when the news finally came.

I had waited twenty years for Irmgard to die. And then I waited for Hans to do the same. In neither case did I desire or control the outcome. But in neither case did I want to be left out of the picture.

I had rushed to Hans's side that first September, hurrying to the emergency room and then spending all daylight hours in the hospital for a week. I sprang into action again in July of the following year, when he was found unresponsive. And in his final crisis, although the phone call caught me unawares, the coil inside me sprang once more and flung me into the fray just as quickly as before. It gave me no time for thought, only for action.

I did not pause to consider that there could have been other ways of reacting. That I could have asked the nursing home for an hourly update. That I could have asked his friends to stay with him in my stead. That hopping on the first flight to Philadelphia wasn't the only alternative.

For me it *was* the only alternative. *I'm his daughter. He might need me. I will rush to his aid.*

And where did I get that from—the instinct to drop everything and go? Who taught me that when I was young? I didn't pause to reflect on this until after everything was over and I was returning to Massachusetts.

It was Hans.

He'd done it for me innumerable times. No matter our disagreements or personality conflicts, I always counted on Hans in an emergency.

"Your car won't start? Just hold on. I'll be over in ten minutes."

"You're not feeling well? I'll just put a lid on this paint can and come get you."

"You need some food?"

"You need my help?"

"You need me?"

"I'm coming."

And his friends confirmed this. "When the cat got stuck on the roof and I was scared to climb the ladder, I called your father." Or, "When the hospital called to say my biopsy results had come back, I couldn't face going alone. I called your father." And, "Who did I call when Bob had a seizure and fell down, blocking the front door while I was out? I panicked and called your father."

Help others when they need it. Not because you're looking for some secondary gratification. Not necessarily because you yearn to be needed. But simply because that's part of being a good human being. Perhaps the most important part. And this part of Hans had become part of me.

And yet . . . there's another side to the end of Hans's struggle.

I had spent almost forty months living Hans's life for him, carrying on my shoulders the weight of his upcoming death alongside his ongoing life. And during all that time I had felt abandoned by the not quite dead Hans in a way I had never felt abandoned by my quite dead mother.

After Irmgard died, I easily imagined her spirit. The essence of her personality reassuringly lived on inside me. She became a conversational companion in my head when I had to make decisions. I sometimes heard her voice admonishing me to be more careful or not to take uncalculated risks. But throughout the period of Hans's dementia, I felt deserted. My former father inhabited neither my mind nor the real world. And none of the transient images of him, the vague outlines I conjured, ever spoke one word of comfort to me.

In my head, Irmgard could talk up a storm. "Never make close friends at the office, because you never know when office politics could change. Always sleep before making a major decision. It's not a good idea to compare yourself to others. Save at least ten percent of your income. Don't eat sugar for breakfast . . ." Irmgard came through loud and clear whenever I wanted her, and sometimes even when I didn't. The phantom mother who never stopped watching and worrying. She lived on inside me, and I never felt completely without her.

The impaired Hans, on the other hand, was completely hopeless as a parent in this respect. He could no longer give me much advice in real life, and I certainly did not want to lean on the person he had become. But he was also miserably incompetent as a spiritual presence. Somehow, his living self prevented my psyche from creating anything in his image. I had nothing but brief, mute, ineffectual visions of him. Having lost him in real life as a source of support, I lost him in my fantasy life as well. What a nightmare, to be deserted by him in both body and spirit.

When Hans died, the weight that had come crashing down on my shoulders lifted. For the first few days I felt a physical reaction. My body experienced a freedom that had not existed before. In addition, now that the impaired Hans was dead, my brain released the healthy, loving, and supportive Hans from my mental prison. Suddenly, before the plane ride back to Massachusetts, Hans stood beside me in the security line.

"Keep breathing. You're too stressed. Relax," he admonished. "And for goodness' sake, smile!"

This vision said familiar things, but I was shocked. *Hans is back now? Just like Irmgard?* But it made sense. After his body was gone, I no longer had to concentrate on the ill-but-living Hans. The memories of my healthy father could once again keep me company.

Despite this improvement, the past forty months had taken a hard toll on me, and initially I reacted in anger. For so long, I had ignored many of my own needs to maintain my focus on my disabled father. Now that his life was over, I grieved for what I had disregarded in myself, for what I had lost in valuing his requirements over my own. I resented having given so much up.

My anger felt perplexingly familiar: I had also been furious with my mother. I had succeeded in smothering my needs in relation to Irmgard's. It gradually dawned on me that I had repeated this mistake with Hans as well. With Hans in his dependent state, our relationship admitted no reciprocity, only imbalance. I had poured all my energy into caring for him without remembering to care for myself. I had felt as though I had no choice, that I had to spend an inordinate amount of time obsessed with Hans.

Had that really been the case?

DURING HIS LAST NIGHT, when the first dose of morphine finally arrived to lessen Hans's discomfort, I relaxed somewhat. Now it will get easier for him. And yet half an hour later, he seemed as uncomfortable as before.

I went to find the nurse.

"The doctor only ordered ten milligrams," she explained. "But he's a big guy. I'll give him another ten, and then we can see what happens."

With that second dose, Hans finally began to slip away—not from life, but from the conscious experience of his distress. His grip on my hand gradually loosened. His breathing eased.

Then, in his last aware moments, Hans used his remaining energy to move his hand. He placed his thumb on top of mine and began, almost imperceptibly slowly and gently, to stroke me. The thumb moved with unhurried deliberation, caressing me lightly. Twice it returned to its starting point to retrace its tender path. Then he lifted his hand from mine and placed it gingerly on his own thigh. There it remained, unmoving, until he died.

Hans's quintessential characteristic shone through in those last gestures. What he expressly wanted to convey by stroking my hand, I am not sure. *Thank you.* Or *Don't worry.* Or *I love you.* There are many possibilities. But no matter the message, he was thinking about *me*. The morphine had eased his suffering enough to make room for Tina in our relationship once again.

My mother loved me, but at the very end of her life, she could only concentrate on herself and her own needs. In order to die, she needed to separate from everything that would still be alive when she was not.

In order for Hans to die, he needed the exact opposite. He needed to hold on to what would continue to live and breathe and love. He made his final communication about me. About us. He embraced the comfort of a shared love and a shared experience. He embraced our connection.

Acknowledgments

This book describes events that made me grateful to have had the support of many generous and caring individuals. I wish to thank especially the following people, who helped in various ways with its completion: Cynthia Bisman, Cliff Carle, Patsy R. Cobb, Nicole Cobb-Moore, Tom Cole, Booth Gardner, Ursel Hofmeister, Barbara Hruda, Vittorio Maio, Beverly Booth McCauley, Nancy and Mac Robinson, Brenda Smith, and Nona Smolko. In addition, the entire team at Vanderbilt, including Michael Ames and Ed Huddleston, has been fantastic.

Antje Hofmeister (known as "Lucy" in the story), who has shared my life as my best friend and as a de facto member of my family, provided invaluable constructive criticism. More than anyone else, she knew me, my parents, and the details of what transpired. Throughout the many iterations of the manuscript, she encouraged me to explore, in a stronger, more realistic light, hidden layers of connection and meaning I avoided or did not recognize. Without her as a sounding board, I would understand so much less of myself than I do, and I would have written so much less of a story.

And Ron Strickland, the husband with whom I feel overjoyed to share my life, provided inspiration in countless ways. As a writer, he advised. As a critic, he edited. As a friend, he supported. As a calmer personality, he guided. And always, as my partner, he waited patiently as I moved through my past and into our present.